AF730835

THE MARY FRANCES FIRST AID BOOK

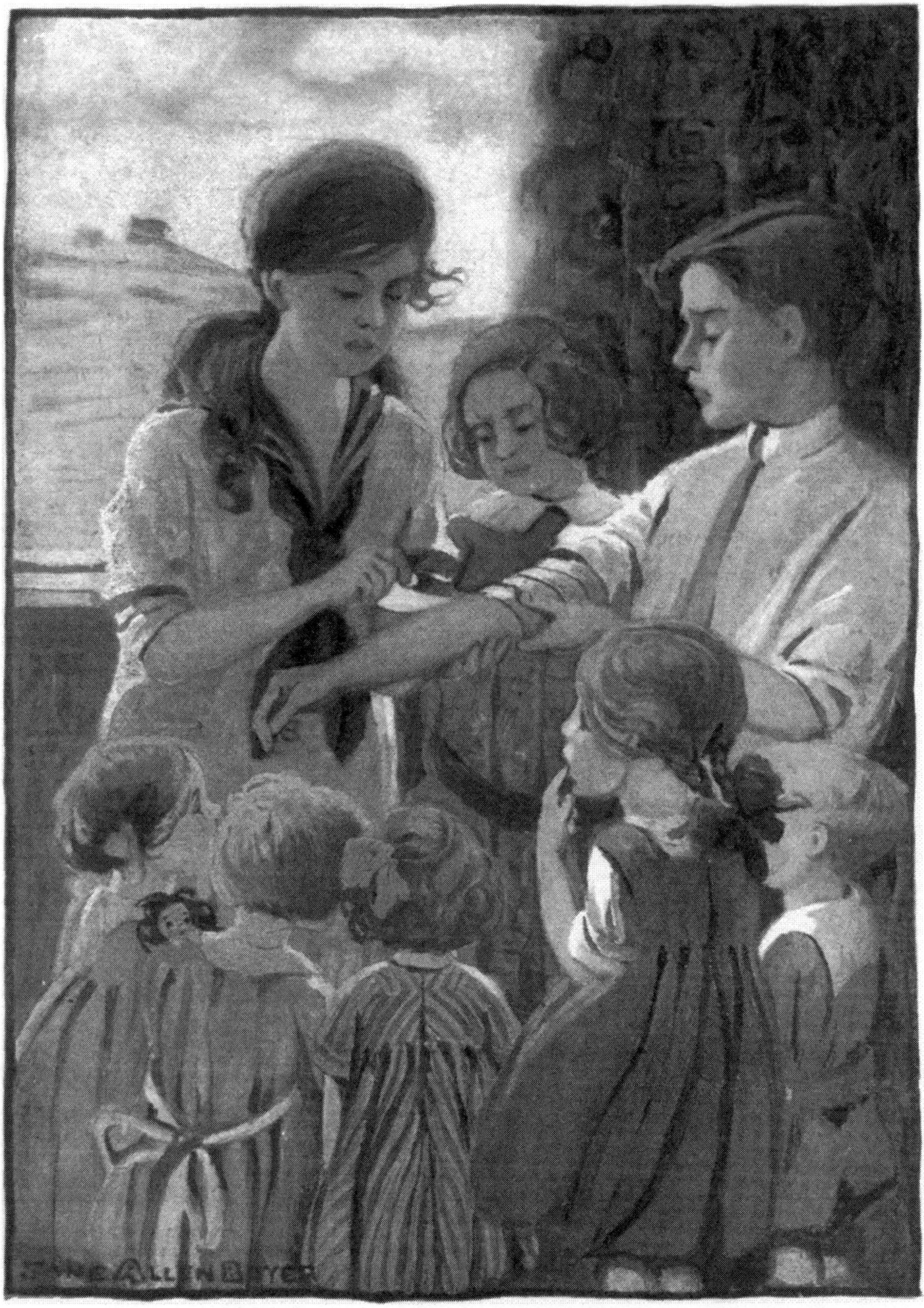

Mary Frances Puts Her First Aid Knowledge into Practice.

THE MARY FRANCES
FIRST AID BOOK

WITH READY REFERENCE LIST OF ORDINARY ACCIDENTS AND ILLNESSES AND APPROVED HOME REMEDIES

By

JANE EAYRE FRYER

Illustrations By

JANE ALLEN BOYER

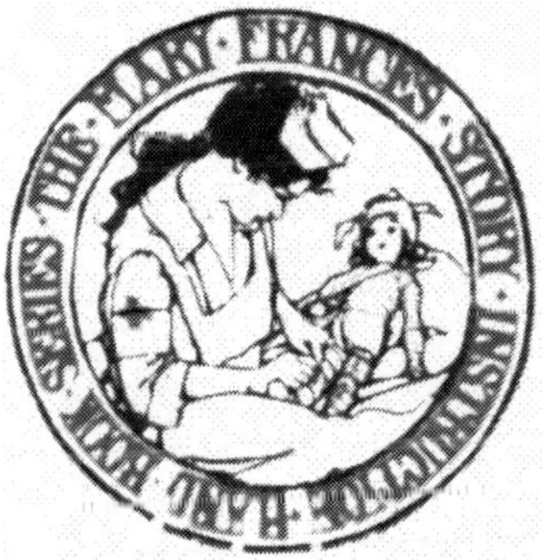

NEW WEST PRESS

ISBN 978-1-64965-280-5

New West Press
Henderson, NV 89052
www.nwwst com

Ordering Information:
Special discounts are available on quantity purchases by corporations, associations, educators, and others. For details, contact the publisher at the listed address below.

U.S. trade bookstores and wholesalers: Please contact New West Press:

Tel: (480) 648-1061; or email: contact@nwwst.com

PREPAREDNESS

THIS book is for every boy and girl who hopes to render first-aid to the sick or injured—in time of peace—in time of war—at all times in the service of

OUR COUNTRY

PREFACE

THIS book is more than a story to inspire children with a desire to relieve suffering; it is a simplified and handy reference book, telling what to do in cases of accident or illness. In no sense is it intended to take the place of the physician. The first principle of first-aid cannot too often be repeated—*when in doubt, send for the doctor.*

Especial thanks are due to E. A. Y. Schellenger, M.D., member Surgical Staff, Cooper Hospital, Camden, N. J., for his great assistance in verifying and revising the medical and first-aid instructions given herein; and to Constance Cooper Crichton, Instructor of First Aid Classes, New Jersey Women's Division National Preparedness, whose helpful criticism and suggestions have been invaluable.

Jane Eayre Fryer

MERCHANTVILLE, N. J.

CONTENTS

CHARACTERS

HOSPITAL STAFF

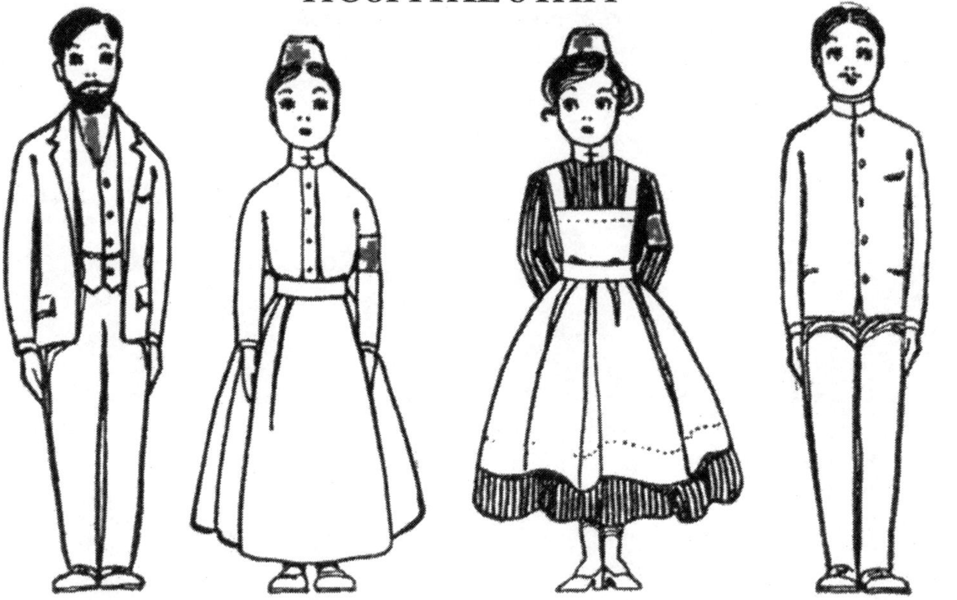

Doctor Surecure
Resident Physician

Miss Bossem
Head Nurse

Miss Helpem (Mary Frances)
Assistant Nurse

Doctor Quickenquack
Interne Physician

POLICE OFFICERS

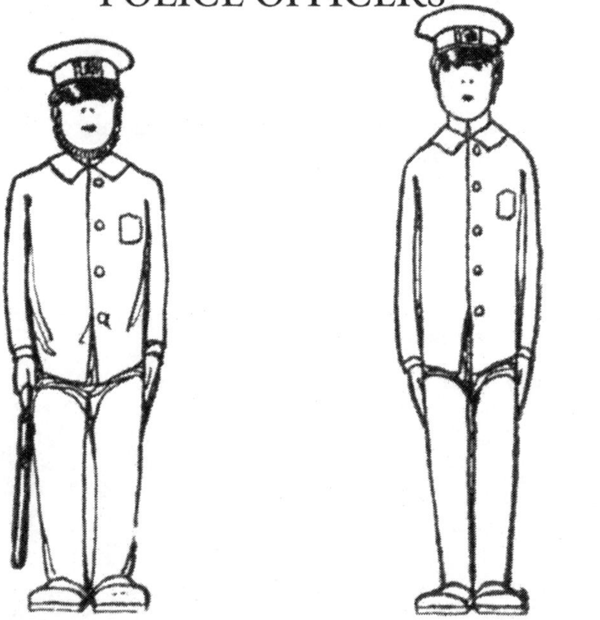

Officer Arrestem
Chief of Police

Officer McStoppem
Assitant Chief of Police

PATIENTS

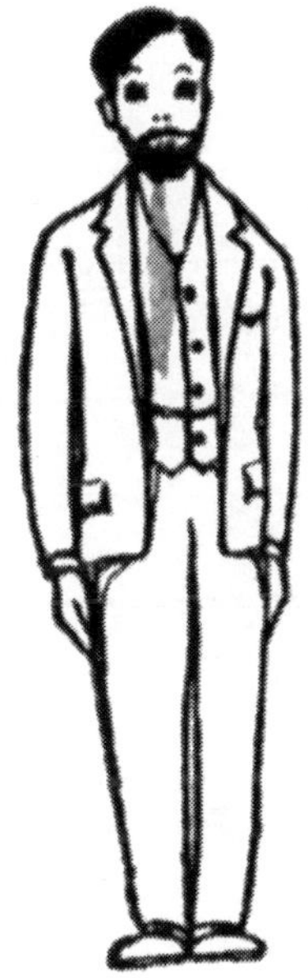

HESA BRAVE
Private Brave's Father

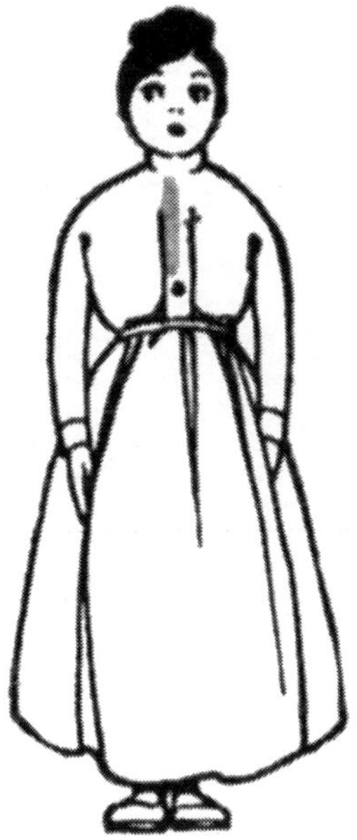

MRS. BRAVE
Private Brave's Mother

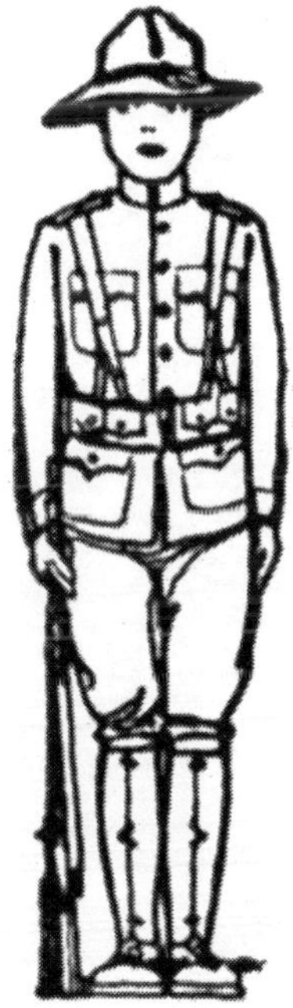

IMA BRAVE
Private Brave
U. S. Army

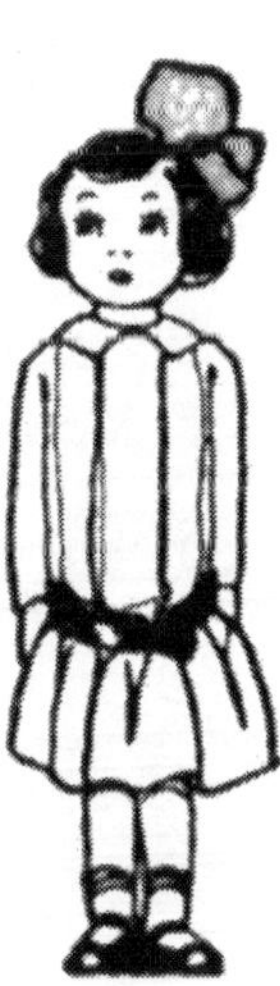

SOAMI BRAVE
Private Brave's
Little Sister

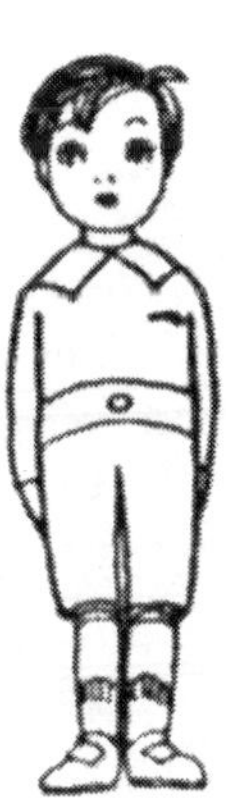

IBEE BRAVE
Private Brave's
Little Brother

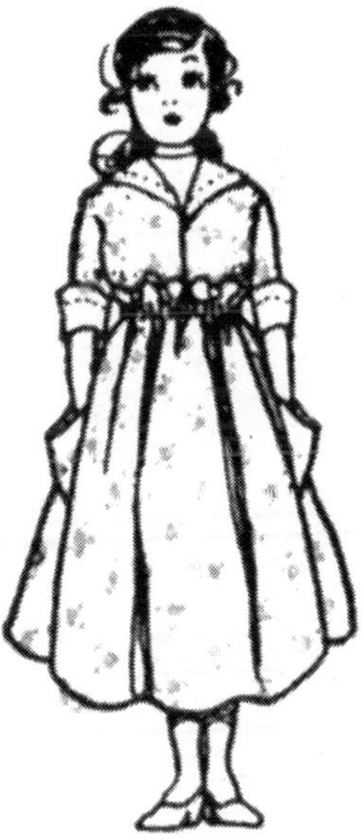

IBEE BRAVE
Private Brave's
Big Sister

CHAPTER I

OFF TO MEXICO

THE Head Nurse, Miss Bossem, rushed out of the Dolls' Hospital toward the children. "You're late, Miss Helpem," she called to Mary Frances. "Go right on duty rolling bandages for the soldiers who start for Mexico to-day. The troop-train leaves at two-thirty. Hurry, now, or you won't get them to the station on time."

Then, turning to Billy, "Get the ambulance ready immediately," she commanded, and Billy disappeared into the garage.

. . . . . .

You see, Mary Frances finished the course in First Aid Nursing with the Red Cross Preparedness Class just before her birthday. Being very proud of her newly acquired knowledge, she wanted to show Billy how much she had learned.

When Billy promised her any favor she could think of as a birthday present, Mary Frances joyfully asked him to spend a whole day at the Dolls' Hospital in the playroom, pretending they were little kiddies again—that she was Miss Helpem, the assistant nurse, and that Billy was the ambulance driver. To keep his promise, Billy consented.

Just as they stepped into the playroom door, they seemed to grow smaller and smaller, until they were no bigger than the dolls themselves.

Now, go on with the story and see what happened.

. . . . . .

Promptly at two-fifteen, Miss Helpem arrived at the station with an ambulance full of bandages, and just in time to see the Brave family bidding good-bye to Private Ima Brave. All the family were there, even Michael, the big bulldog. Private Brave was among the last of the soldiers to board the little train.

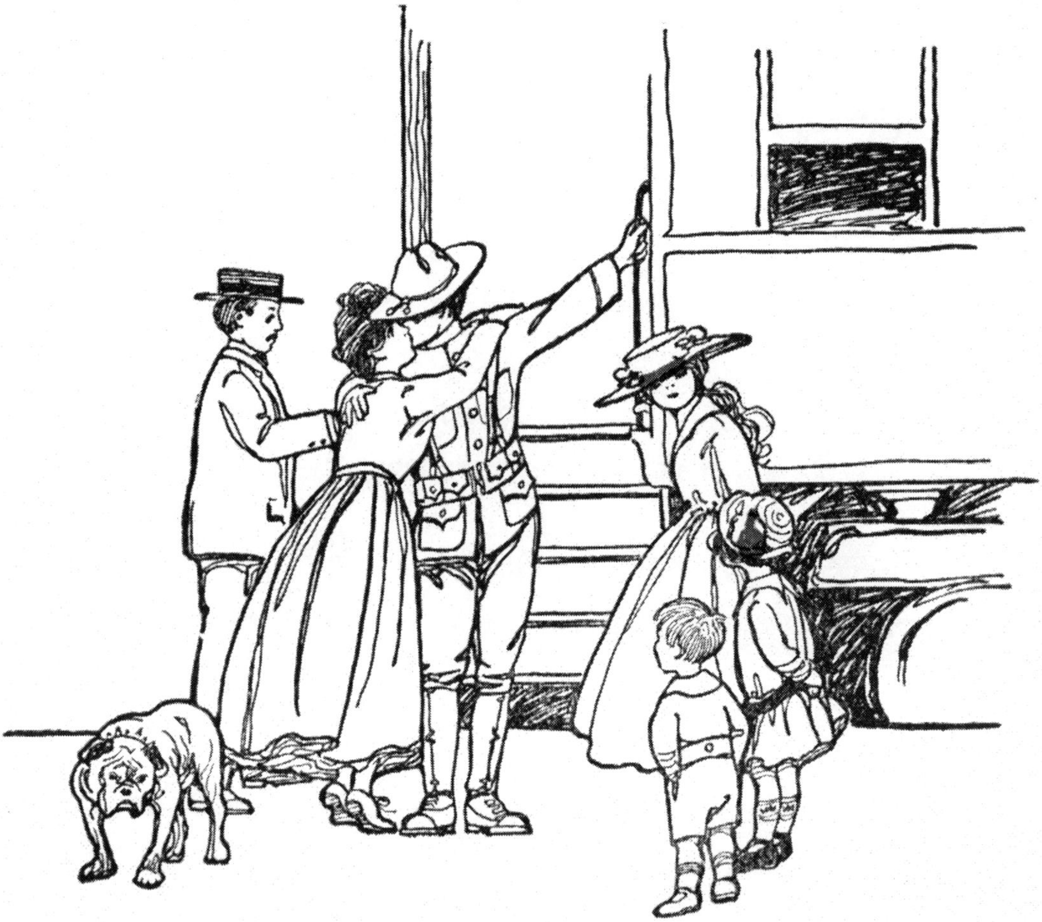

"ALWAYS CARRY THIS WITH YOU"

"You'll write from New York, dear," begged his mother, kissing him for the twentieth time, and slipping a little American Red Cross first-aid outfit in his hand. "Always carry this with you, and remember how your mother loves you."

"And you'll send me picture postcards from everywhere, won't you?" begged little Ibee Brave, standing on tip-toe to get a better view of his tall, straight brother.

"There's a speck of dust on your uniform," fussed Soami, his little sister, as she brushed him with her handkerchief.

Private Brave smiled. "We're not on dress parade, little sister," he said. "It's good that khaki doesn't show the dust, for it's a dusty country we're going to."

"'It's a long, long way to Mexico, it's a long way to go,'" began little Ibee; but at that moment the engine whistled, and his father clasped Private Brave's hand.

"I am proud of my son," was all he said.

"And I, of my brother," Shesa, his big sister, added, with tears in her eyes.

One more whistle, and the little train started down the playroom railroad track.

"We'll bring the limousine nearer the station," said Mr. Brave, taking Mrs. Brave's arm and walking away.

"Father and Mother don't want anyone to talk with them just now," said Shesa.

"I don't see why. Gee, I wish I was big enough to go," said little Ibee, as he watched the train until the last car turned a curve in the track.

"You'd make a fine soldier, wouldn't you," laughed Soami, "when you're afraid to go upstairs in the dark."

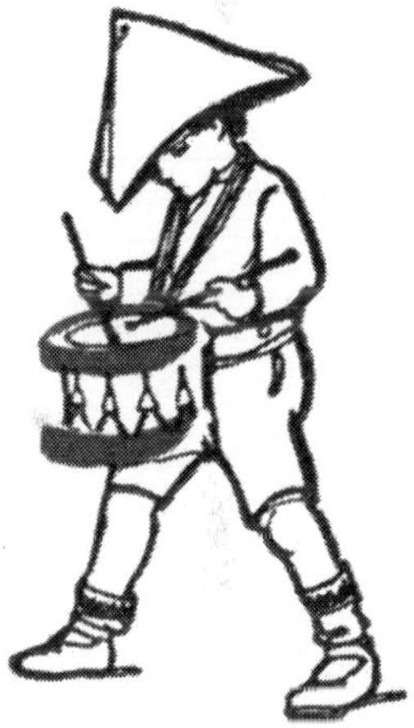

'MY! HE CAN DRUM BRAVELY!"

"Only sometimes," answered Ibee; "only when the wind blows hard and when it's not moonlight—and then, not often."

"Why, Soami, Ibee is real brave," said Shesa. "Don't you remember how you were afraid to go down cellar to get some jam last night and Ibee would have gone, if father hadn't made you go?"

"Yes, and father stood on the landing the whole time you were gone, too, Miss," declared Ibee triumphantly.

"Yes, that's so," acknowledged Soami. "I guess Ibee would make a good soldier—especially a drummer boy. My! he can drum bravely! Did you hear him yesterday, Shesa?"

"Indeed I did," laughed the sister.

"Yes," continued Soami, mischievously, "don't you remember the verses about—

'A little man bought him a big bass drum,
        Boom-tid-dee-ah-da-boom!
"Who knows," said he, "When a war might come?
        Boom-tid-dee-ah-da-boom!
I'm not at all frightened you understand,
But if I am called to fight for my land,
I want to be ready to play in the band.
        Boom-tid-dee-ah-da-boom!'"

"Come, children," said their father, driving up, "here's the car. Hop in."

CHAPTER II

THE SPEEDERS' ACCIDENT

THE shrill sound of a policeman's whistle cut the air three times, but the dollsmobile sped on faster than ever.

"I couldn't catch them at all, at all," reported the little thin sub-officer, McStoppem, at headquarters.

"Bring my motorcycle, McStoppem," ordered Chief Arrestem.

"All right, sir," nodded Officer McStoppem, bringing out the wonderful little toy. "If you take the cross-cut road toward Sandpile Village, you'll catch them. The number is—here it is, I wrote it down—1492. You can easily remember it—the year Columbus made 'preparedness' necessary."

"Cut out your chatter, McStoppem, and follow me in a hurry," directed the chief, as he kicked the pedal of the motorcycle to start the engine. "Hand me the paper," and, snatching it, was off.

"The chief'll get 'em O.K.," muttered Officer McStoppem to himself, as he watched the long line of dust and smoke in the wake of the little motorcycle.

. . . . . .

Just as Chief Arrestem came into the cross-roads leading to Sandpile Village, the runaway automobile flew past.

"By Jiminy, I don't wonder McStoppem couldn't catch them," he said under his breath, as he put on still more speed. "That man's lost control of his car, and unless I'm mistaken there'll be an accident when he comes to that dangerous turn in the road where that big rocking chair stands."

Meanwhile everybody in the dollsmobile was trying not to be frightened.

"Can't you slow down a little, Father?" asked Mrs. Brave.

"The brakes won't hold," panted Mr. Brave, forcing both brakes on with all his might. "This is dreadful!"

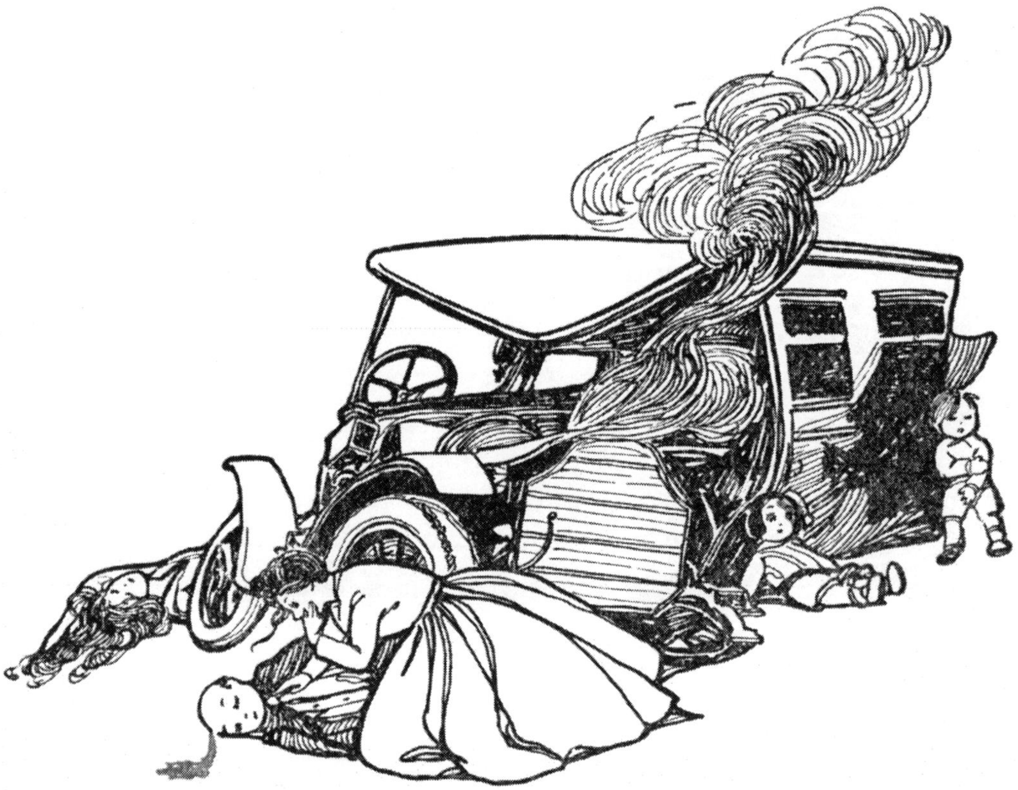

"OH, THE ENGINE'S ON FIRE!"

"Gee whiz!" exclaimed little Ibee, looking out the rear window. "Here comes the motor police. He'll arrest us for speeding."

"Oh, mercy, we're coming to Rocking Hill road," gasped Shesa. "Father, do turn off the power!"

But Shesa spoke too late, and kerr-smash! kerr-bang! kerr-plunk! went the dollsmobile right into the rockers of the rocking chair, turning "turtle" twice, and breaking the beautiful glass windows to pieces. Out of the broken radiator the boiling hot water poured over poor Mrs. Brave's arm where she lay just as she was thrown.

"Oh, the engine's on fire!" shrieked little Soami, "and I'm burning to death!"

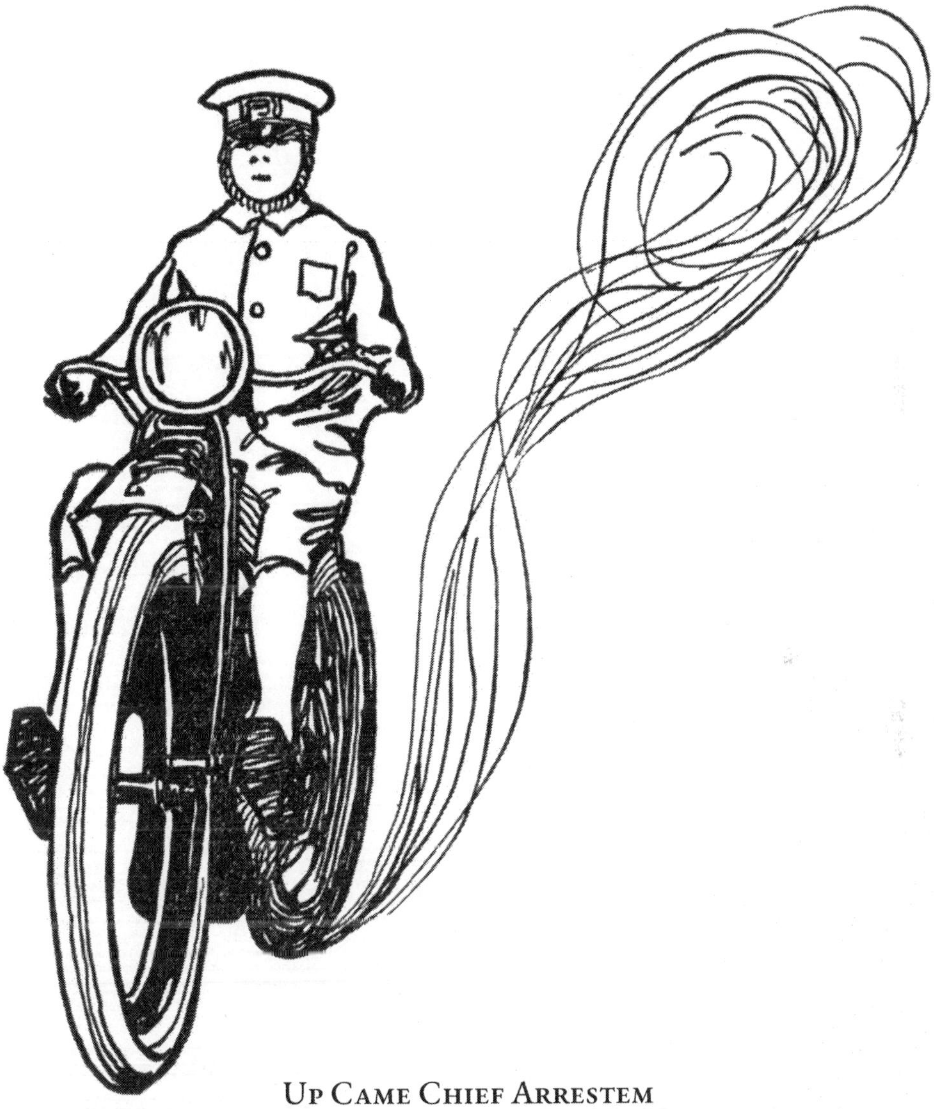

Up Came Chief Arrestem

"Father, Father," called little Ibee, "come get me out! I'm fast under the car! Come get me out, please! Oh, I'll be burned to death! Father, oh, my arm hurts! Oh, I can't move my arm!"

The mother managed to get up when she heard the children call.

"Where's your father? Oh, where is he?" she cried, and going to the other side of the car, she saw poor Mr. Brave lying amidst a heap of broken glass and wheels and gears. From his head ran a little stream of blood.

"Oh, he's dead!" she sobbed, but just then he gave a little groan. "Oh, my dear husband," she exclaimed, "tell me you're not dead! Tell me you're not dead!" she begged, unmindful of her own arm.

"I'm dead, Mother," groaned little Soami. "I just know I'm dead with pain."

"Well, I'm not!" said little Ibee, "and even though my arm hurts so, I'm going to try to go for help if I can get out from under this car."

"My, that's so!" exclaimed the mother. "I myself forgot to be brave. I'll go for help."

But just as she spoke, up came Chief Arrestem.

"I saw it all, madam," he said, "and I stopped to telephone to the hospital for the ambulance."

"Oh, don't 'rest us, please," begged little Ibee. "Please, Mr. Officer, don't arrest us. We weren't speeding. Father couldn't make the brakes hold!"

"Don't you worry, little chap," replied Chief Arrestem. "I won't arrest any of you. Here comes Officer McStoppem on his motorcycle, just as I told him to, and in a minute we'll have you all out from under."

"Never mind about me," said Ibee. "Please get poor Soami out. She's dead, I think."

"Quick, McStoppem," called the chief, "help throw sand on this car to put out the fire!"

It took about ten seconds for the two officers to put the fire out, and even before that, they heard the honk! honk! of the ambulance.

"Here comes the ambulance!" cried Chief Arrestem. "Now, with the driver's help, we'll soon be able to lift this car."

CHAPTER III

FIRST AID TO THE INJURED

NOW, all at once," directed Chief Arrestem. "One, two, three!" and the two officers and the two ambulance men lifted the dollsmobile high up over to the other side of the road.

"Well, friends," said Officer Arrestem, "if there's nothing more we can do, we'll return to our duty."

"Nothing more, thank you," the head nurse answered.

The driver had quickly smothered the flames of little Soami's frock by using the automobile robes.

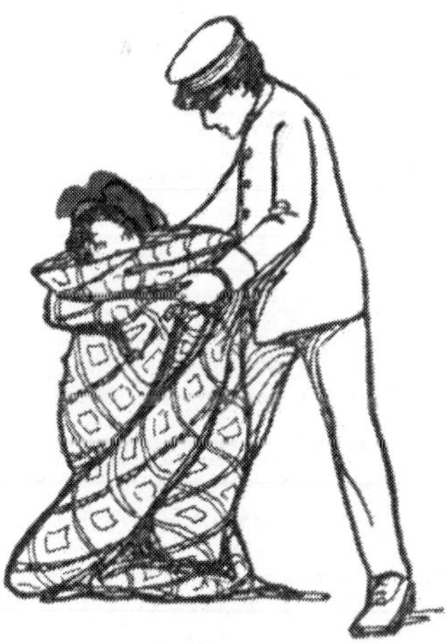

SMOTHERED THE FLAMES OF LITTLE SOAMI'S FROCK

"Oh, my goodness!" shrieked Mrs. Brave, "where's Shesa? I wonder where my dear daughter is! Where is she? Where can she be?" she kept on asking, crying hysterically.

"Hush! quiet yourself!" commanded the assistant nurse, who came in the ambulance. "We found your daughter a few moments ago where she was thrown. She had fainted, but she is all right now."

"Oh, sit her up; don't let her lie there!" exclaimed the mother.

"Indeed, you must keep quiet," said the nurse, "or we cannot do anything for anybody. It is better for her to lie down than to sit up."

"I'd keep quiet if I knew what to do! Every woman and man, too, ought to know."

"Yes," replied the nurse, "every person ought to know something about first aid to the injured." She and the other nurse were busily directing the orderly and driver of the ambulance in every movement, giving them explicit directions.

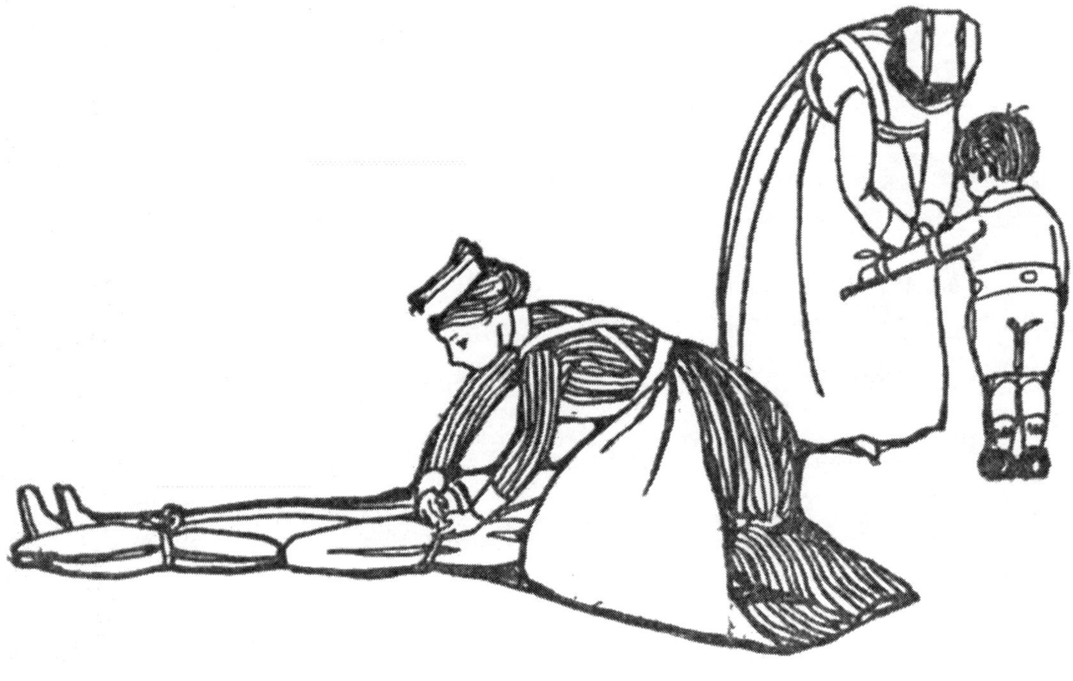

THEY ATTENDED THE MOST DANGEROUSLY INJURED FIRST

They attended the most dangerously injured first, stopping the bleeding (hemorrhage) of Mr. Brave's head and bandaging a dressing in place. They applied soothing carron oil to the burns on little Soami's arms and legs.

They bandaged temporary splints to little Ibee's broken arm, and, since Mrs. Brave's scalds were not serious, they attended her last.

Under Mr. Brave's broken leg they placed pillows to make him more comfortable.

"If I'd only remembered to turn off the power this never would have happened," he muttered. "How foolish of me!"

"There would never be any accidents to speak of," said the assistant nurse, soothingly, "if everybody did everything right, you know."

"If everybody just kept his head cool," said Mr. Brave, as he tried to move his position, but fell back with a groan.

"Give him a half-teaspoon of aromatic spirit of ammonia, Miss Helpem," said Miss Bossem, who was engaged in spreading the stretcher.

"Now, everyone ready to lift this patient," she directed, as she and the driver and orderly knelt on one knee beside Shesa, and Miss Helpem took her position on the opposite side of the stretcher. As the three lifted Shesa, Miss Helpem carefully held the stretcher in place, and afterward helped carry the patient to the ambulance. Next they carried the two children, using a stretcher for little Ibee, and making a two-handed seat for Soami. (A "sedan chair," you know—the kind you play with at school.)

"I'm sorry neither doctor could leave the operating room to come, Miss Helpem," remarked Miss Bossem, to her assistant, who was Mary Frances, you remember. "If you will wait here with these two patients," (they were Mrs. and Mr. Brave) "I will return with either Doctor Surecure or Doctor Quickenquack."

"Oh, why can't you take my dear husband along?" begged Mrs. Brave. "He's awfully hurt! awfully!"

"Please explain to her, Miss Helpem," said Miss Bossem, getting into the ambulance, "that it is far better to wait for the doctor to attend a broken leg than to attempt to place it in splints—unless it is absolutely necessary to move the patient."

Miss Helpem turned to Mrs. Brave, who was by this time quite exhausted, and after explaining the situation, treated her, as she had all the others, for—

SHOCK

Cause:

A severe injury, or even the sight of one, will often cause intense nervousness, which is very weakening. This is especially true if the patient is suffering from severe bleeding. *Check the bleeding before treating for shock.*

Shock differs from fainting. The patient's face becomes pale and the skin cold, the pupils of the eyes large.

What to do:

1. Send for the doctor.
2. Place patient on back with head low to allow plenty of blood to enter head.
3. Give hot water or hot coffee, or one-half teaspoonful aromatic spirit of ammonia in a quarter of a tumbler of water.
4. Hold smelling salts to the nose.
5. Do not excite by trying to remove clothing unless absolutely necessary, but keep patient warm by use of hot-water bottles and blankets, etc.
6. Cover patient. Rub limbs toward body.
7. Do not give whiskey or any other form of alcohol, if any other stimulant can be found—and never whiskey in case of hemorrhage (severe bleeding).

CHAPTER IV

AT THE DOLLS' HOSPITAL

IN a short time Mrs. Brave began to feel better, and, by the time the ambulance returned, was able to stir about.

"Let us have a look at this broken leg," said Doctor Quickenquack, examining Mr. Brave. "Ahem! I think, Miss Bossem, after all, we would better use—

First-Aid Treatment for Broken Leg

(*See Reference List*)

Place pillows under the leg to make it more comfortable, but do not move the patient before the doctor comes, unless absolutely necessary. If necessary to move, place a board or an umbrella, one on each side of the leg, and tie in place, (or tie both legs together if it seems advisable) using bands of muslin, handkerchiefs, or *triangular bandages.

"After we have Mr. Brave in the hospital, we'll put that leg in the right kind of splints and bandages," remarked the doctor, as he and the driver and orderly placed him on the stretcher. "You'll be running a race like a boy in a few weeks," he continued encouragingly as he seated himself beside the patient in the ambulance, and the nurse helped Mrs. Brave to a place.

*Triangular bandages are described in Chapter XIII

"Like a tortoise, I'm thinking," said Mr. Brave, trying to joke above the pain, for oh, how his broken leg did ache.

Clang! clang! clang—clang! sounded the ambulance gong, and in less than a few minutes they were at the Dolls' Hospital.

. . . . . .

The next, morning little Ibee came into his father's room, where his mother was sitting beside the bed with her scalded arm nicely dressed and bandaged.

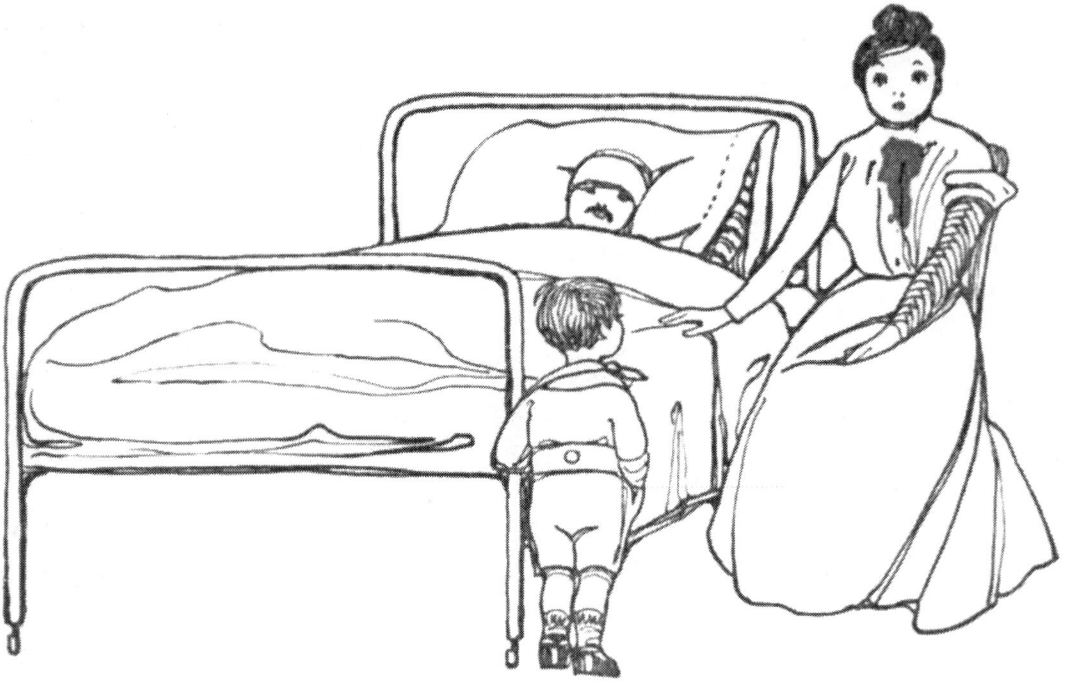

HIS MOTHER WAS SITTING BESIDE THE BED

"I'm going to be a doctor," he announced proudly, after bidding his parents good-morning. "This is a dandy place! There aren't any private rooms for Soami or me, so we're each in a ward, and there's a fellow in the men's ward all done up in bandages. I just wish you could see him! I got Doctor Quickenquack to tell me what kinds they all were and I can't remember all of them, but I know he said something about triangular and spiral and figure-of-eight bandages. My, that fellow looks fine! He has a broken arm and a broken leg and a dislocated shoulder and a fractured jaw, and his bandages are swell! He did the whole thing by sliding off his barn roof last Sunday when he was putting shingles on it. He says it's a judgment—whatever that is."

"Well, for pity's sake," exclaimed his mother, "Ibee, how you talk! Do take a breath!"

"Hello, everybody!" said little Soami, running in. "How's father? Shesa's fine, Miss Helpem told me. No bones broken except one finger. Shesa's asleep now, and her finger's bandaged beautifully!"

"Father's just about as well as can be expected, dear," answered their father. "And very thankful none of us are hurt worse."

"I don't know," said Ibee, shaking his head. "Even though my arm aches so, I'd have liked to have had something worth while; for instance, a compound fracture of the thigh. Father's was only a simple fracture. In a compound fracture the broken bone often comes through the skin, I heard the head nurse say to one of the assistants."

"Well, sir," said his father, "if you had this, you'd find it was enough!"

"Why, what's the matter with the boy? Is he crazy?" exclaimed his mother. "As though we hadn't all had trouble enough!"

"I don't think he's crazy," said Soami. "There's a girl in our ward who has a broken nose, and it looks too interesting for anything to see the nurse dress it! I want to be a nurse when I grow up! Just think how many people one can help! Why, if it hadn't been for the nurses, perhaps we might—nearly all be dead!"

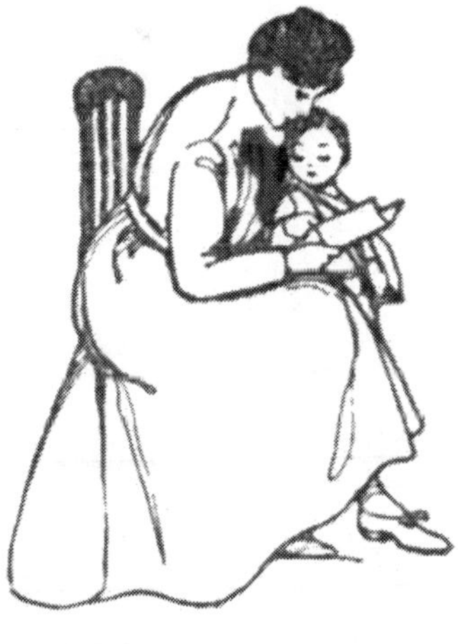

"Read it out Loud!"

"Indeed we might," agreed their mother. "I don't know whether you'll be a doctor, Ibee, or whether Soami will be a nurse, but I do know that I'm going to ask Miss Bossem if a class cannot be formed in our neighborhood in which we can all learn how to render first-aid to the injured."

"Good for you, Mother," said Shesa, coming in at that moment, and kissing her father. "I've just been talking with Miss Helpem, and she has explained how to join the Preparedness Movement, so that if we should have war right in our own land, or serious accidents, we could help care for the wounded or injured."

"That brings my dear Ima to mind. Oh, I do hope we'll get a letter to-day," said her mother.

"Here's a postcard just received for Master Ibee Brave," said a nurse, coming along with the mail.

"From Ima!" said Ibee. "It's from New York," looking at the postmark.

"Read it out loud!" cried his mother. "Let us all hear how the dear boy is."

Ibee read:

Dear Folks:

New York never looked better to us than as we left for the front—but who wouldn't be brave for the sake of the red, white and blue? Will write mother a long letter as soon as time permits.

As ever,

Ima Brave.

"Now, isn't that brave?" exclaimed his mother. "He's as brave as Teddy Roosevelt!"

"It's wonderful to belong to such a brave family," said Miss Helpem, who came in just then to renew the dressing on Mr. Brave's head.

CHAPTER V

THE REAL CROSS NURSES

COME," she added, "this excitement will never do for Mr. Brave. Everybody leave the room, and everybody go to bed and take a nap."

"I don't want to," began Ibee. "I want—" but at that moment, Miss Bossem, who was passing, came into the room.

"Why, what does this mean?" she asked crisply, gazing around. "How does it happen, Miss Helpem, that all these people are in the invalid's room? Everyone who comes in must have permission."

"Well, I am surprised!" exclaimed Mrs. Brave. "As though I'd have to ask permission!"

"Well," replied Miss Bossem, in a very decided manner, "everybody who stays in this hospital must obey the rules. Miss Helpem, will you kindly see that the children are put to bed, and I will take Mrs. Brave to her room."

"I'm no child," began Mrs. Brave, "I'm an older woman than you, and I've had——"

"Do you intend to risk your husband's life any further?" asked Miss Bossem, lifting her eyebrows and speaking in a low, icy tone.

"Poor wife—" began Mr. Brave.

"See!" said Miss Bossem. "He's already too excited to rest tonight without some medicine."

"Oh, dear," whispered Mrs. Brave, "I'm so sorry!" Then aloud: "Miss Nurse, I'm real tired. I think I need a nap. Good-bye, dear, I'm going to my room—you take a nap, too."

"Well," said Miss Bossem to Miss Helpem, "I did succeed in making Mrs. Brave see how dangerous it was to excite the patient, but my, I don't like to be so cross!"

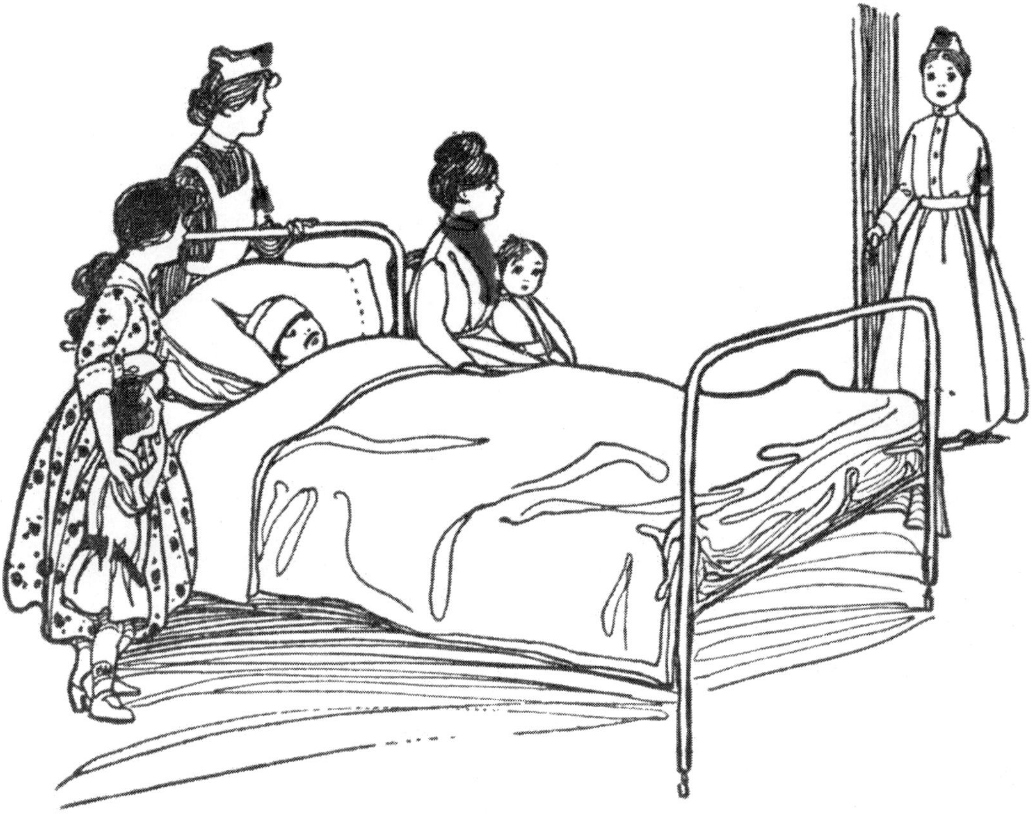

"WHY, WHAT DOES THIS MEAN?"

"I just had to be firm with the children, too," replied the assistant nurse. "But Shesa's a dear, and has extraordinary good sense. She is going to form a class in Red Cross first-aid work."

"Yes, and we'll give the instructions," said Miss Bossem; "that is, if you are willing."

"Of course," answered Miss Helpem, "but what I meant to tell you is that Miss Shesa is going to form a class for children."

"What a lovely idea!" exclaimed Miss Bossem, passing on into the clinic.

. . . . . .

"Doctor, I'm getting quite tired of being here," complained little Ibee to Doctor Surecure, when he met him in the corridor one day about three weeks later. "Of course it's dandy to see so many banged-up people, but I'm nearly well. My arm aches only on rainy days, and I can wiggle my fingers fine."

"Good," smiled the doctor. "I'm thinking myself that we'll be parting with some of the Brave family soon. Your mother and sisters are to leave us Saturday."

"Can't I go, too, Doctor? Can't I?" begged the little boy.

"Why, that's a pretty way to talk," replied the doctor. "Don't you like us?"

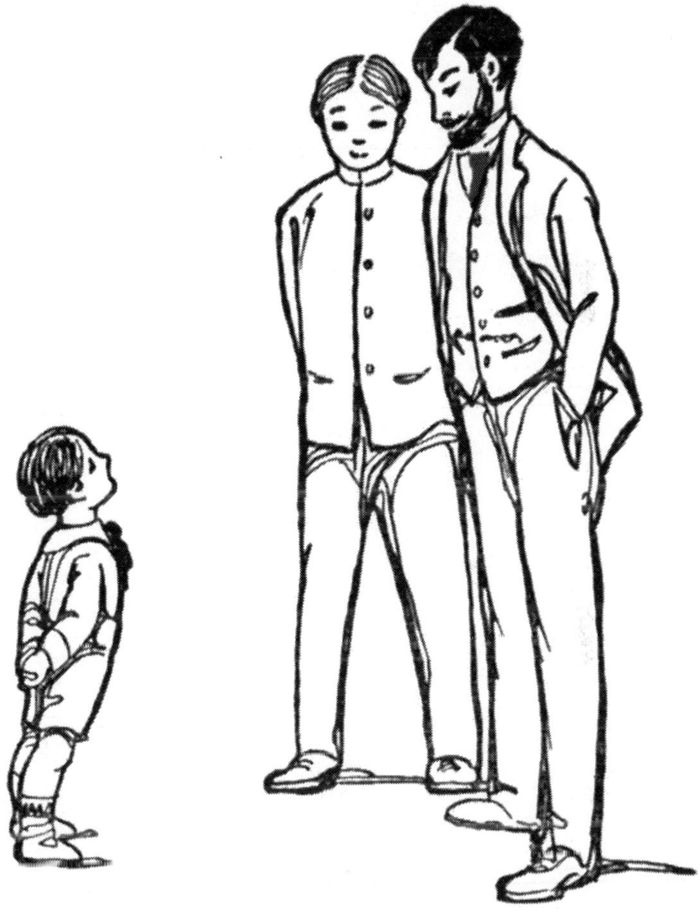

"CAN'T I GO, TOO, DOCTOR?"

"Oh, sure," said Ibee, "but the fellows miss me a lot, you know."

"Why, what will your poor father do without any of you?" teased Doctor Quickenquack, who happened to be passing.

"Oh, I'll come see him every day," said Ibee. "He'll love to hear all about home. Can't I go?"

"We'll think it over," said Doctor Quickenquack.

"And if we do decide to let you go," added Doctor Surecure, "you must promise not to try to take off your bandage."

"Oh, I promise," said Ibee. "Doctor Quickenquack said that if I let my arm be in it long enough, I'd be able to play baseball again: and besides, I want to show it to the fellows."

"But you'll not pitch ball for some time to come, young man," laughed the doctor.

So Mrs. Brave and the children were soon in their own home, leaving poor Mr. Brave in the hospital. By the time Mr. Brave was able to return, walking with a crutch, they had formed three first-aid classes. Mrs. Brave's was for grown-up ladies, and of this Shesa was a member. Shesa herself, with Soami and Ibee's help, had formed two others; one for Boy Scouts, and one for Camp Fire Girls.

CHAPTER VI

LESSONS IN FIRST AID

"MISS HELPEM," said the head nurse to her assistant, "how would it be for you to take charge of Miss Brave's children's classes, with her help, of course? If you think well of that arrangement, I will take the adult class, and leave the children's instructions to you."

"Nothing could please me better, Miss Bossem," answered Mary Frances (I mean, Miss Helpem). "I dearly love dolls—oh, I meant to say, children."

Miss Bossem laughed. "Perhaps you'll grow up some day," she teased.

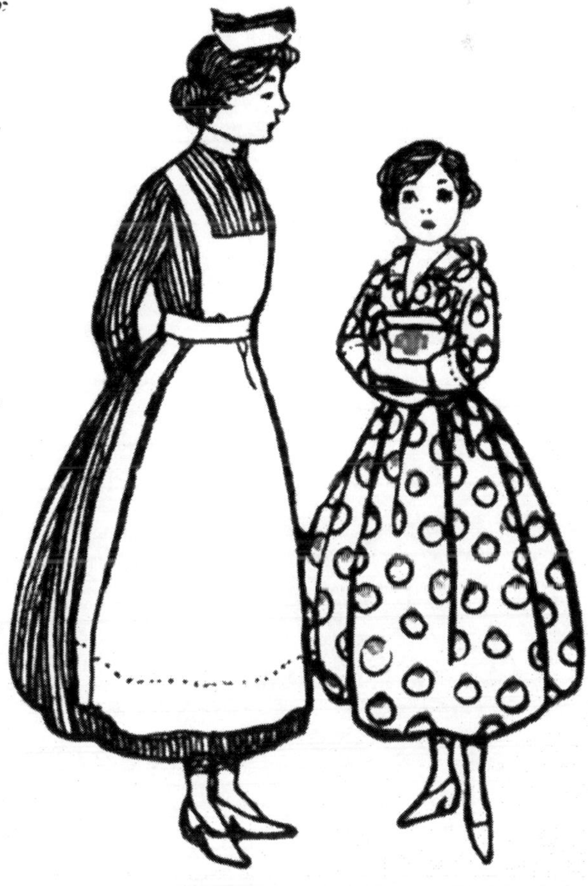

MISS HELPEM WAS TALKING WITH SHESA BRAVE.

. . . . . .

"How would you like to assist me with the children's lessons?"

Miss Helpem was Talking with Shesa Brave

"Oh, do you really think I would be able to do that?" asked Shesa, delighted.

"Yes," answered the nurse, "Miss Bossem and I feel quite certain you can be a great help in showing the boys and girls what you learn in the women's class."

"I never felt so proud in my life!" declared the young girl, hugging her first-aid kit close in her arms.

. . . . . .

So it came about that when Mary Frances' dolls gathered together for their lessons, it was Mary Frances herself dressed in the spotless white uniform, with the red cross on the arm and cap, of the American Red Cross Society, who gave their—

FIRST LESSON

IN

FIRST AID TO THE INJURED

"Good morning, children," she began. "We will imagine all kinds of troubles and accidents this morning, and we will not be a bit gloomy over them, for our thoughts will all be on how we can help the sick and hurt people."

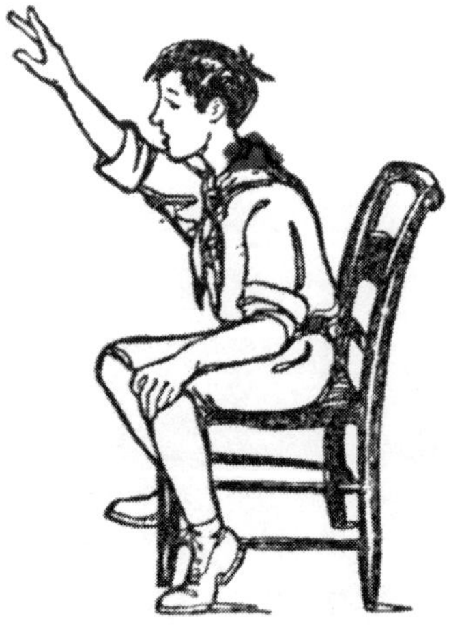

"PLEASE, MISS HELPEM, CAN'T I BE THE SOLDIER?"

"Please, Miss Helpem, can't I be the soldier?" begged Ibee Brave.

"And can't I pretend to drive the field ambulance?" asked little Jack.

"And can't I be run over?" asked another boy.

"Mercy, children," exclaimed the nurse, "please wait for an explanation—and in the next lesson, I'll assign you all something to do. Now, ready with your note-books and pencils to take down the list of articles needed for the medicine closet. You will learn what they are to be used for later. Keep the list and show it to your parents when you get home. Now write as I dictate:

MEDICINE CLOSET

In every home there should be a certain closet or shelf high above little children's reach, where the medicines and articles needed in emergencies are kept. Among these should be found, plainly labeled, the following:*

1. Tincture of Iodine.
2. Aromatic Spirit of Ammonia.
3. Boric Acid Powder.
4. Stearate of Zinc.
5. Pure Alcohol.
6. Lime Water.
7. Carron Oil.
8. Epsom Salt.
9. Soda Mint and Pepsin Tablets.
10. Baking Soda.
11. Household Ammonia.
12. Adhesive (Zinc Oxide) Plaster.
13. Tube Vaseline.
14. Capsicum Vaseline.
15. Peroxide of Hydrogen.
16. Castor Oil.
17. Witch Hazel.
18. Essence of Ginger.
19. Syrup of Ipecac.
20. Spirit of Camphor.
21. Sweet Spirit of Nitre.
22. Boric Acid Ointment.
23. Powdered Alum.
24. Borax.
25. Spiced Syrup of Rhubarb.
26. Picric Acid Gauze.
27. Aromatic Smelling Salts.
28. Oil of Cloves.
29. Normal Salt Solution.
30. Powdered Mustard.
31. Essence of Peppermint.
32. Tincture of Arnica.
33. Oil of Turpentine.
34. Aseptic Absorbent Cotton.
35. Sterile Gauze.
36. Triangular Bandages.
37. Roller Bandages.
38. Rubber Ear Syringe.
39. Fountain Syringe.
40. Measuring Glass.
41. Eye Dropper.
42. Hot Water Bottle.

*The full list of remedies, with explanatory notes, is given in the Ready Reference List at the end of this book.

The children wrote very quietly and listened attentively to what Miss Helpem told them about being prepared for Ordinary Household Accidents, such as cuts, burns, scalds, bruises, stings, etc.

. . . . . .

"Children," beamed Miss Helpem as they finished writing the list, "I never dreamed you could be so interested. Why, not one of you has been inattentive! Now, as a reward, I shall show you how—

To Make a Sanitary Drinking Cup from Any Piece of Clean Paper***

(****Editor's Note*: The original book had a removable page with folding instructions on how to make a paper cup capable of holding water. There are many website and video tutorials online with similar instructions.)

CHAPTER VII

SAFETY FIRST

"WE girls get our second lesson before you boys do!" declared little Soami to her brother Ibee at the lunch table the next day.

"I bet you don't have as much fun as we do!" answered Ibee.

"What is the next lesson about?" asked their father.

"It's about Safety First," replied Ibee. "I know that."

"Yes," agreed Soami, "but," glancing at the clock, "I'll be late to class if I don't hurry. Mother, will you excuse me?"

Her mother nodded and smiled, and Soami left hastily.

. . . . . .

"Well, girls," began Miss Helpem, "to-day we have a more serious time, for we're going to learn, in Lesson II, What to Do in Case of Slight Cuts and Pin Pricks; Slight Burns and Scalds; Frost Bites.

"Now, as you know, almost every accident could be avoided if we thought ahead far enough; if we did not let the knife or needle slip; if we did not allow little children to carry scalding hot water or lighted lamps, or to play with matches; if we looked up and down the street before crossing. Yes, almost all accidents are avoidable if we think far enough ahead—if we think 'Safety First.'"

Miss Helpem paused.

"All ordinary everyday accidents," she went on, "if treated rightly, will give but slight trouble; but if not treated rightly may bring much suffering to the victim, and even cause 'blood poisoning' and death.

"So you see how necessary it is to understand 'What to Do.'

"Now, these serious dangers do not come from the slight accidents themselves, but because of uncleanliness."

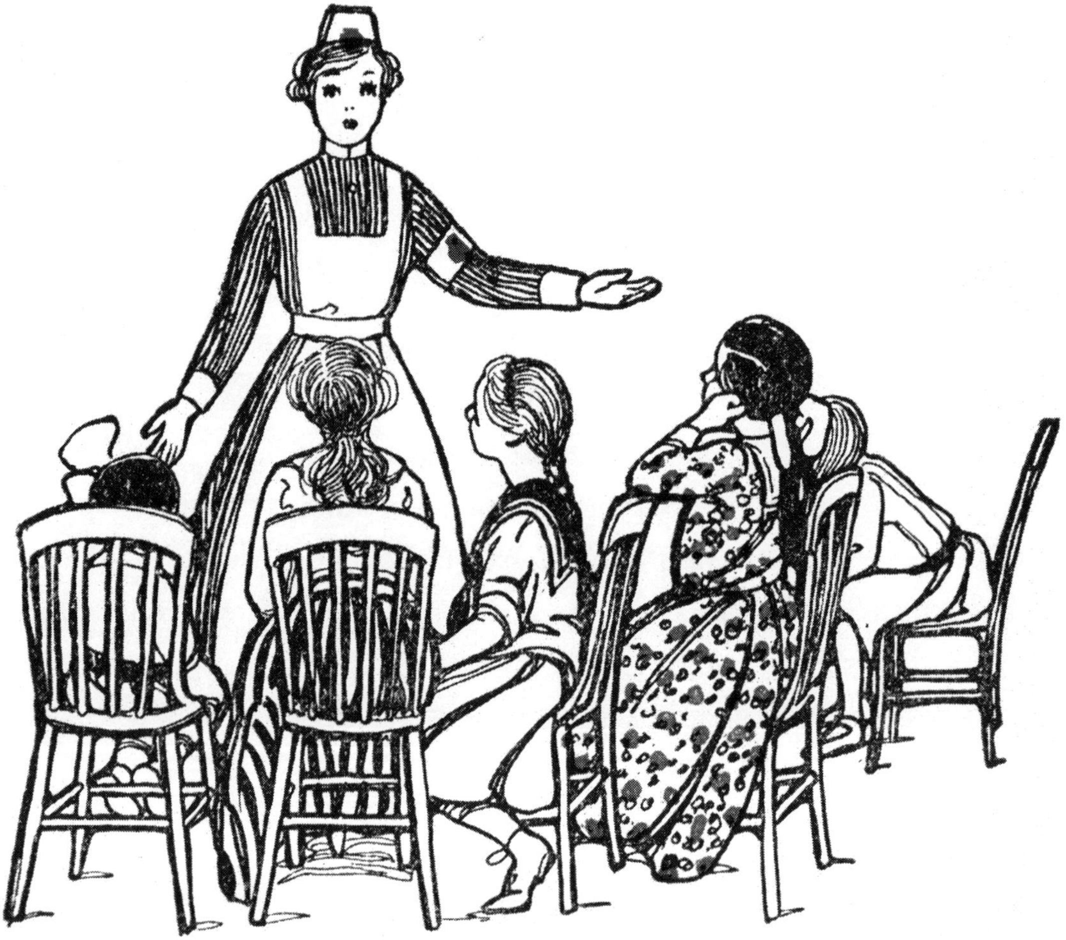

"WELL, GIRLS, TO-DAY WE HAVE A MORE SERIOUS TIME"

Again the assistant nurse paused, and she could not help smiling at the look of astonishment on the faces of her girl dolls.

"It is true, girls," she continued; "cleanliness is the rarest thing in the world, and I will tell you why: because everywhere about us, in the dust, in the air, on our clothing, on our hands, in standing water, on the floor, on the ground—everywhere, even though we cannot see them, are

Germs

These little living particles are too small to be seen without a microscope, but they cause more disease and deaths than any of the big animals you are afraid of—like lions or bears or tigers. They make great deep sores out of little cuts, and prevent wounds from healing. So you can readily understand how necessary it is to keep all materials which touch broken skin perfectly clean, and they cannot be clean if touched by the hands. Neither is any material clean which has come in contact with dust.

Understanding this, your aim will be to keep germs out of any wound. If you do not have a first-aid outfit, you should have on hand a small package of sterile gauze.* Sterile means perfectly free from germs. Any cloth which has been washed and ironed is quite safe, however, if it has not been used. You see, heat kills germs. Use next to the wound the surface which has been folded inside.

Do not think that every germ does evil, for some germs are good—just as some people are bad and some are good. Indeed, we depend for some kinds of food upon the action of certain good germs. Among such foods are cheese and vinegar.

The disease germs which we dread most in cases of wounds are the germs of blood-poisoning and lockjaw (or tetanus). They are everywhere about us, in standing water, air, dust. They cannot do a bit of harm to the outside of the body, if the skin is unbroken—no more than a fly can do to the armor of some old knight. But if they can enter where the skin is broken, they begin to do all kinds of harm, which sometimes results in months of suffering from "infected" wounds, and sometimes finally causes the patient to lose a leg or an arm—or perhaps to die.

"We have spent a great deal of time on the subject of germs, children," continued Miss Helpem, "because unless you really understand how necessary cleanliness is, you may not be particular to have clean materials."

"And clean hands," suggested Soami.

"Yes," smiled the nurse, "Soami has noticed the nurses at the hospital washing their hands for five minutes in order to have them truly clean before attending to a dressing on a patient."

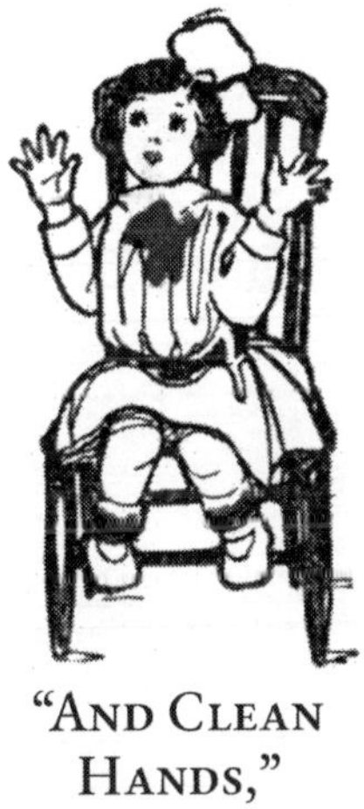
"And Clean Hands," Suggested Soami

*Sterile gauze is cheesecloth which has been so treated that it is free of germs and is very absorbent. It is sold at all drug stores. It should be kept closely wrapped, and the surface should never be touched with the hands before it is placed on a wound.

If you do not have sterile gauze, keep old linen or cotton cloth (which has been well washed and ironed) in glass jars, which have been boiled and dried in the air without wiping.

The little girl looked around proudly upon the class.

"Can't we begin the first-aid games now?" asked one of the group.

"Not yet," the nurse shook her head. "Wait, please, until you have learned what to do for—

SLIGHT CUTS AND PIN PRICKS

The bleeding from a slight cut is never very severe and will generally stop of itself in a short time. It is best to let a slight cut bleed a little, as the bleeding carries away the germs which may have been on the edge of the knife or whatever caused the wound.

Treatment:

Touch slight cute with tincture of iodine;* or with alcohol; or vinegar and water, half and half; or salt and water, a half teaspoonful of salt to a cup of water.

Wrap with clean gauze.

In cases of severe hemorrhage (bleeding) send immediately for a doctor. Stop bleeding by using pressure above or below wound, or by bandaging a gauze compress on the wound.

Never give whiskey or alcohol in any form. It makes hemorrhages worse. See Reference List.

BURNS AND SCALDS

(See Reference List)

Apply carron oil. See List of Medicines.

If carron oil is not at hand, use any dressing† to cover surface to keep out the air—as lard, butter, olive oil—or sprinkle with baking soda, or cover with white of egg, or with a paste made of starch or flour and water. Also spread on compress† some of the same remedy that has been applied to the burn. Hold compress in place with a loose bandage.

Solution of bicarbonate of soda (baking soda) made by dissolving as much soda as

*Soldiers on active service carry iodine to be applied to wounds immediately, if possible—to kill germs. Iodine is a poison if swallowed, so be careful not to leave it within the reach of small children.

†Important Note.—Dressings are everything applied to a wounded or sore surface. A compress is the dressing which is placed directly upon the wound. It is usually made of clean new gauze. A bandage is the dressing which holds the compress (or other dressings) in place.

Compresses are used to—

1. Hold medication in place.
2. Protect sore place.
3. Stop bleeding.

possible in hot water (about one teaspoonful to a cup) is particularly relieving to scalds. Dip cloths into this and apply to the burned surface. Never remove skin from blisters. If blisters are large, see the doctor.

HOW TO PUT OUT FLAMES

Caution.—If your clothing catches fire, *do not run!* Roll (in a rug, if possible) *on the floor or ground!*

In putting out fire on another person's clothing, use rugs or blankets. In throwing a rug on another person, be careful not to allow your own clothing to catch fire. Let the sufferer lie down and roll. Stand in back of the rug, and throw from the head downward.

If in a burning building, creep to the door on hands and knees to avoid the smoke.

TO AVOID ACCIDENTS FROM FIRE

1. Children should not make bonfires without the aid of older persons.
2. Matches should be kept out of reach of small children.
3. Children should be taught to be careful of open fireplaces.
4. Children should be taught to roll if their clothing catches fire. This would save scores of lives in a year.

Safety First. Look ahead! See the danger before the accident!

FROST BITES

When nose, ears, hands or feet are exposed to intense cold they often become frost-bitten, turning purple at first. If frozen thoroughly, they turn waxy white; then no pain is felt, because the nerves are frozen.

Treatment:

1. Keep patient in cold room.
2. Do not warm frozen parts quickly. Instead, rub with snow or bathe with ice water until a tingling pain is felt; then stop.

If frozen parts are warmed too quickly, "gangrene" may result, or perhaps the sudden heat may cause—

CHILBLAINS

Chilblains are the result of too rapid warming of cold parts, generally feet or fingers. Sometimes for years after being frost-bitten, exposure to severe cold will produce itching and burning, and perhaps swelling and ulcers.

Treatment:

Rub with turpentine or alcohol. The rubbing in itself is excellent. See doctor.

CHAPTER VIII

PRACTICE GAMES

"THAT is all the lecture part of to-day's lesson," smiled Miss Helpem. "Now, for the practice."

She made a gesture toward Shesa Brave, who came forward, and together they lifted before the class the tiny medicine cabinet which Mary Frances' Aunt Maria had given her for her Dolls' Hospital.

"Let me see," said Miss Helpem. "Yes, we have everything here, I believe. Girls, you may all come look."

The dolls—I mean, girls—gathered around the little glass closet and compared the labeled bottles and packages with the list given them in the previous lesson.

They were delighted with the beautiful cleanliness of the closet—its bright glass door and white shelves and shining enamel frame.

"Now," continued Miss Helpem, "please divide into groups of two. That will make five groups. We will play that one girl in each group is the mother, and the other her child. The child has cut her hand while slicing bread. Mothers, what will you do? What will be your first-aid treatment?"

Mary Frances—I mean, Miss Helpem—was delighted with the girls' answers and with the way in which they sought out the iodine bottle, and wrapped the supposed injury with narrow gauze.

"In the next practice game, the 'child' acts as mother and 'mother' as 'child,'" said the assistant nurse. "This time the 'child's' clothing has caught fire from a spark which snapped out of the fireplace."

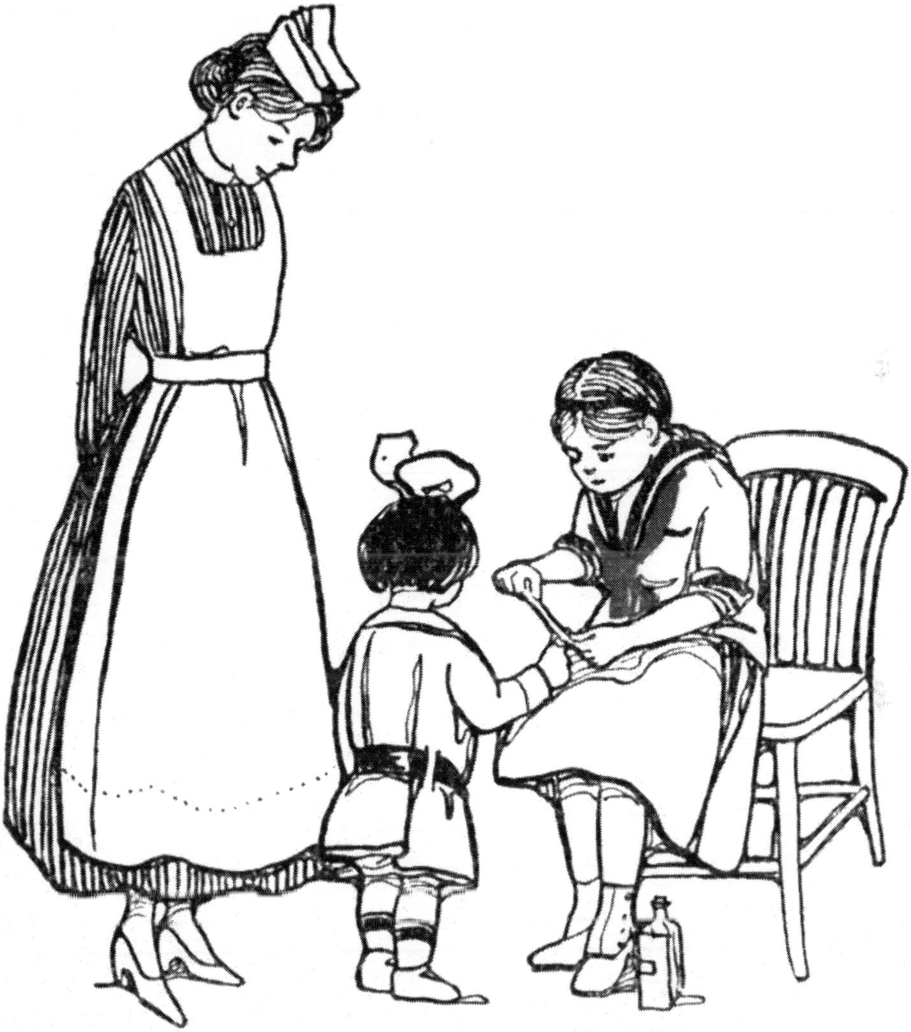

WRAPPED THE SUPPOSED INJURY WITH NARROW GAUZE

The girls laughed.

The nurse smiled. "Girls," she said, "these games may make you feel like laughing, but please keep in mind how serious the real accident would be, and try to learn what to do. You will be so much better able to live useful lives."

You see, Mary Frances didn't quite remember that they were only dolls. Even so, they have served a very useful purpose if they only teach the readers of this book some of their lessons.

"Ready, now, for practice," said the nurse. "Girl No. 2 of each group is to act as a little daughter whose frock has caught fire."

The girls remembered not to run, and "pretended" to smother out the flames.

"That was so well done," said Miss Helpem, "that no one was severely burned, so we'll merely have to treat for slight burns."

The "mother" girl from each group went to Shesa Brave for carron oil, which she applied on gauze compresses to imaginary hurt fingers.

Then they reversed parts again, and played the "child" had frosted her fingers. The "mother" girls rubbed the fingers with imaginary snow, gradually restoring the circulation of the blood in the "frozen" parts.

Throughout all their fun the girls acted in a serious, purposeful manner.

"I'm not so certain that boys would 'play in earnest,'" said Miss Helpem to Shesa.

"I think they would," replied the young girl. "I'm certain Ibee is just as interested as Soami," which pleased the assistant nurse more than I can tell you.

CHAPTER IX

THE HIKERS

THE assistant nurse had very little time for the next lesson in the boys' class, so she gave them only notes in the morning, promising the practice games at four o'clock in the afternoon. After telling them of this plan, she began the lesson.

"Probably you boys have never thought of the fact that the little pipes and larger tubes which carry the blood may be broken under the skin," Miss Helpem said. "When the blood gathers in dark purplish spots underneath the unbroken skin, you have what is called a bruise or contusion.

Bruises (Contusions)

(See Reference List)

"Black and blue" spots which result from bleeding under the skin are caused by falls or blows, or pinching (as in door or window).

Treatment:

Apply cold water or ice wrapped in a cloth, or an ice bag, or bathe with half water and half alcohol, or witch hazel, or arnica.

If an arm or finger, hold up over the head.

If severe, after the pain and swelling have lessened, use hot applications, wringing cloths out of hot water, changing them as they cool, or use a hot-water bag.

For "black eye," bathe with ice-cold water, or use cloths wrung out of water as hot as can be borne.

Massage gently for discoloration.

NOTE.—Never open a blood blister—apply hot water.

SPRAINS

(See Reference List)

should be treated as soon as possible by a physician, but while waiting for the doctor, use cold water applications. If cold water does not relieve the pain in an hour's time, try hot water.

Do not attempt to use the sprained joint.

STINGS AND BITES OF INSECTS

(See Reference List)

For stings of bees and bites of spiders, apply any of the following list:

Mud.
Slice of onion.
Household ammonia.
Paste made of bicarbonate of soda (baking soda).
Spirit of camphor.

Miss Helpem paused. "While we are thinking about insects," she said, "I wish to speak of—

THE FILTHY FLIES

If you could look at the bottom of a fly's foot under the microscope, you would see thousands of the most disgusting germs, particularly of the dreaded typhoid fever.

Please remember that it is far more important to prevent disease than to cure—so do all that you can to keep flies out of the house, out of food, off the baby's bottle and body. Just looking at this picture shows you a little of what must go into baby's mouth after the fly has stolen a bit of baby's breakfast. How many of you promise to do everything you can to reduce the number of flies in this beautiful country of ours—by destroying them and by removing their breeding places, which are in manure piles?"

Every boy's hand shot up.

"Thank you," smiled the assistant nurse. "I can see that the boys of this class are to be real soldiers of health for this entire community."

"Please, Miss Helpem," said Ibee Brave, "there are two more animals I would like to learn something about. One is the mosquito, and the other is fleas."

The boys laughed.

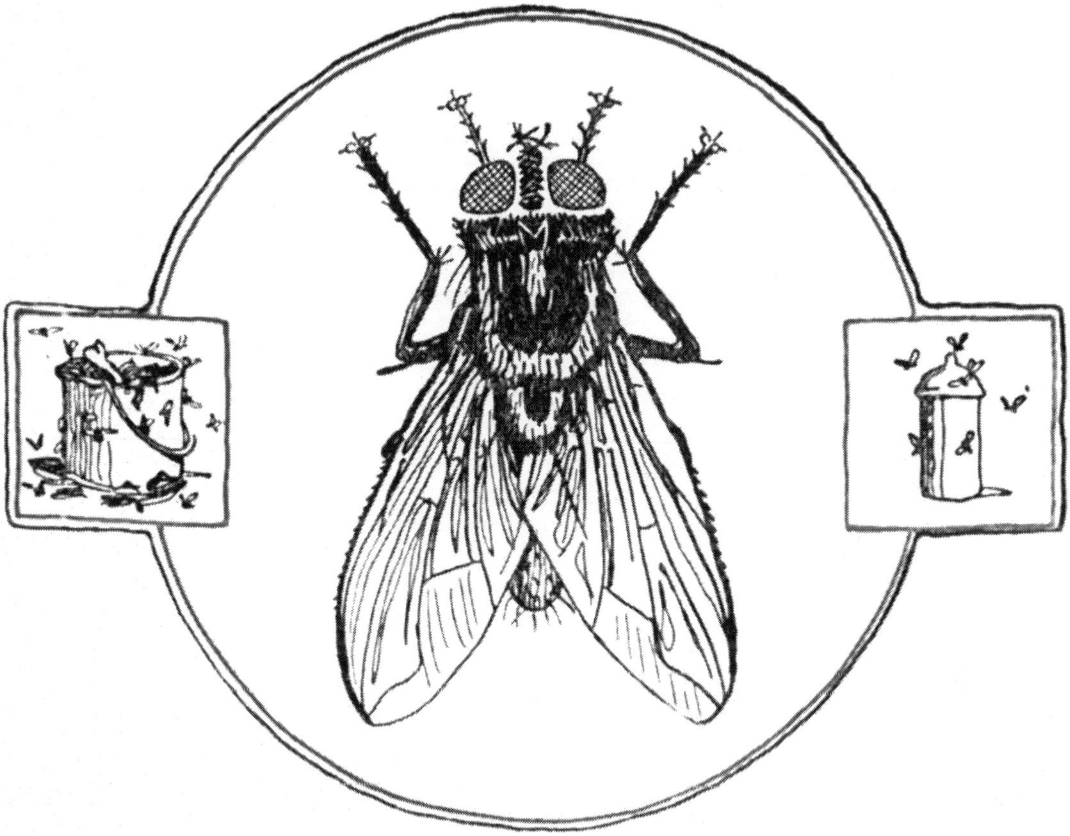

KEEP FLIES OUT OF FOOD, OFF THE BABY'S BOTTLE

"Not animals, Ibee; insects," corrected Miss Helpem. "We will not have time to speak at length of the mosquito, for that would make a whole lesson in itself, but I do want to say that mosquitoes are the cause of some of our worst diseases, for they carry disease germs from one person's blood into another's. To destroy them, kerosene oil should be sprayed or sprinkled or poured on the surface of any stagnant water; for mosquito babies (wigglers) live in stagnant (standing) water. Please remember this: one old tin tomato can half full of water will be an ample amount to supply a whole neighborhood with young mosquitoes in a short time, so overturn any old tins you see, just to help in a good cause."

"Now, Ibee," she continued, after a slight pause, "I will tell you

How to Rid a House of Fleas

Dust naphtha flakes* all over the floors. Leave twenty-four hours, if possible, then sweep up and sprinkle the sweepings with kerosene to destroy the eggs before throwing away.

"I say, fellows," sang out Ibee Brave, after the class was dismissed, "let's go on a hike like any good scouts. Gee, I wish I were twelve years old, so I could be a boy scout!"

"We treat you just as if you were one. Let's go over to the river bank," suggested their patrol leader. At the signal, off they started over the hills of the sand-pile of Mary Frances' playroom, coming at length to Painted River and Looking Glass Lake, on which floated the toy ducks and swans which Mary Frances' little friend Eleanor had given her for a Christmas present.

When they re-assembled at four o'clock, the assistant nurse was surprised at their appearance, for several swollen faces were plastered in blotches of mud.

"We don't need any practice games," commented one of the boys.

"We have had real practical practice," explained their leader.

"I should judge you had," said Miss Helpem, looking over the group. "Do tell me what happened."

"When we left here, we started on a hike to the river," went on the leader, "and after we had rested a little while, we began a game of baseball. Tom Holden was catcher, and somehow when he leaned over to fasten his shoe, bang! the ball went into his eye—an accident, of course."

"At first I thought it had put my eye out," said Tom, "but the fellows used 'first aid' immediately."

*May be bought at drug store, or large department store.

"I never saw a 'black eye' look better," praised the assistant nurse. "You must have had good treatment."

"Next," continued the leader, "I raised a blood blister on my finger, splitting kindling wood for a camp fire. The fellows made some water hot on the fire, and I held my finger in it—but if it hadn't been that we were 'first aiders,' I wouldn't have noticed a little thing like that."

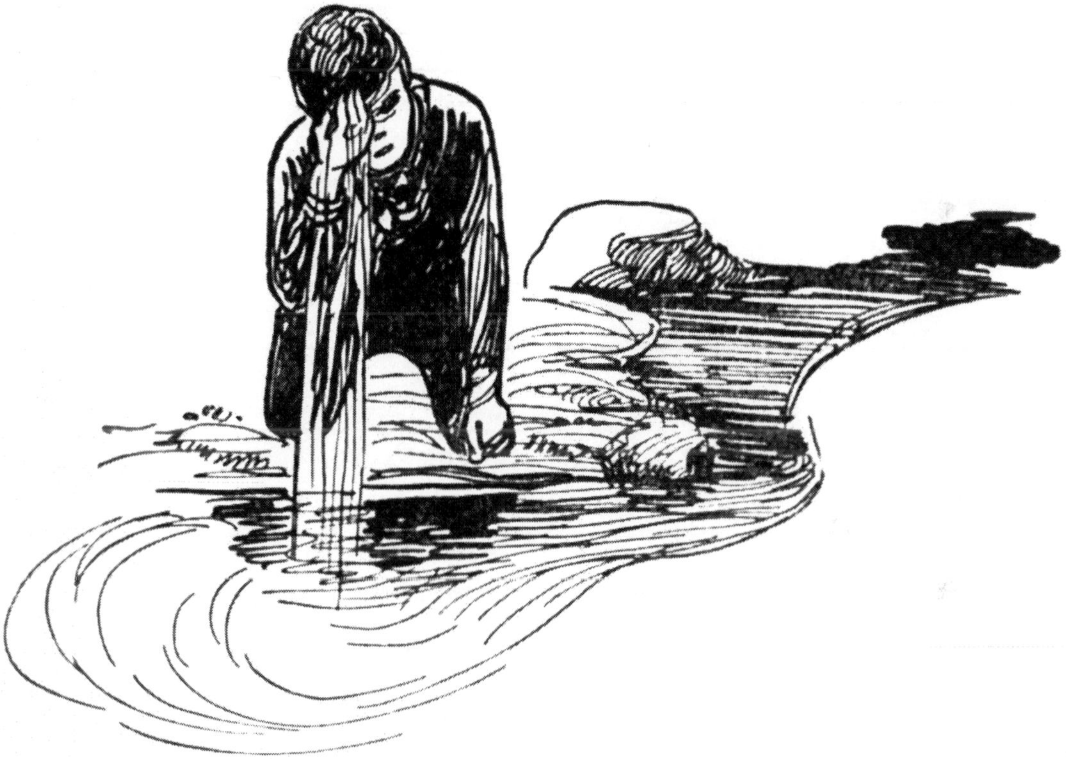

"YOU MUST HAVE HAD GOOD TREATMENT"

"And last of all," said Ibee Brave, "I stepped into a hornets' nest!"

"I can imagine the rest of the story," smiled Miss Helpem. "And I can understand why you haven't clean faces!"

"But you can't imagine how grand it was to know 'what to do,'" protested Ibee Brave through swollen lips.

"Well, boys," said the assistant nurse, "after this day's happenings, I think we

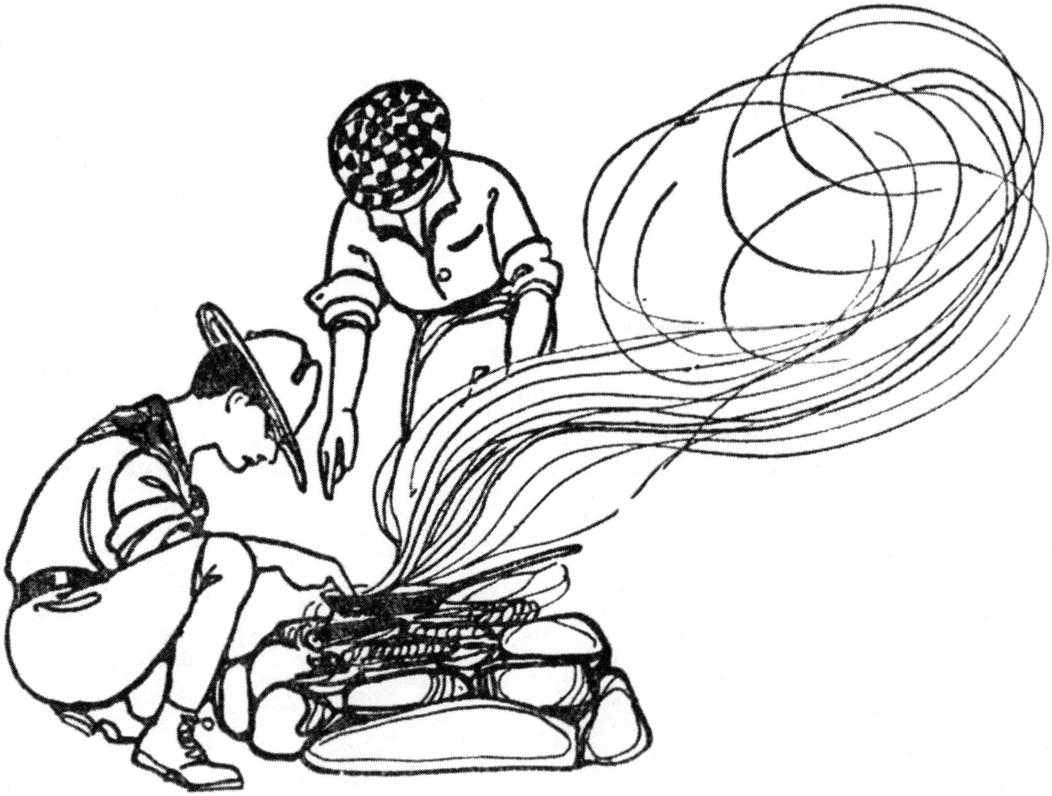

"I HELD MY FINGER IN IT"

will not need any practice games. I'm very glad nothing really serious occurred, and that your first-aid knowledge prevented suffering."

"Say, Miss Helpem, you wouldn't mind not saying anything to the other class about the things that happened, would you? We might just pass it off without much explanation, you know."

"I promise secrecy!" laughed the assistant nurse.

CHAPTER X

ON LOOKING GLASS LAKE

THE boys, however, forgot that Mary Frances' girl dolls were Camp Fire Girls, and "Blue Birds," and that girls as well as boys go on hikes—and meet with mishaps.

The mother of Soami Brave's chum was the Guardian of their Camp Fire. The very afternoon that the boys went hiking, she took the girls of the first-aid class for a boat ride on Looking Glass Lake. They didn't happen to meet any of the boys, however.

The sun shone very brightly into the playroom window, a beam falling radiantly upon Looking Glass Lake and reflecting brightly upon the faces of the happy boating party.

"Isn't this lovely!" sighed Soami, as they drifted under the shade of a Christmas cedar tree which Mary Frances had planted on the edge of the lake.

"Isn't it, though!" said Angie, her little chum; "only isn't the sun hot, Mother!"

"It certainly is, dear," agreed her mother. "I didn't realize, or I would have told you to powder your faces to prevent sunburn."

"Why, Mother!" exclaimed Angie, "you have always disapproved of face powder, and here you are recommending powder!"

"I know," laughed her mother, "but I refer to toilet or talcum powder, a coat of which might prevent sunburn. As it is now, you girls will probably have to ask Miss Helpem's advice."

"Our class meets to-morrow morning," said Soami. "Isn't that good!"

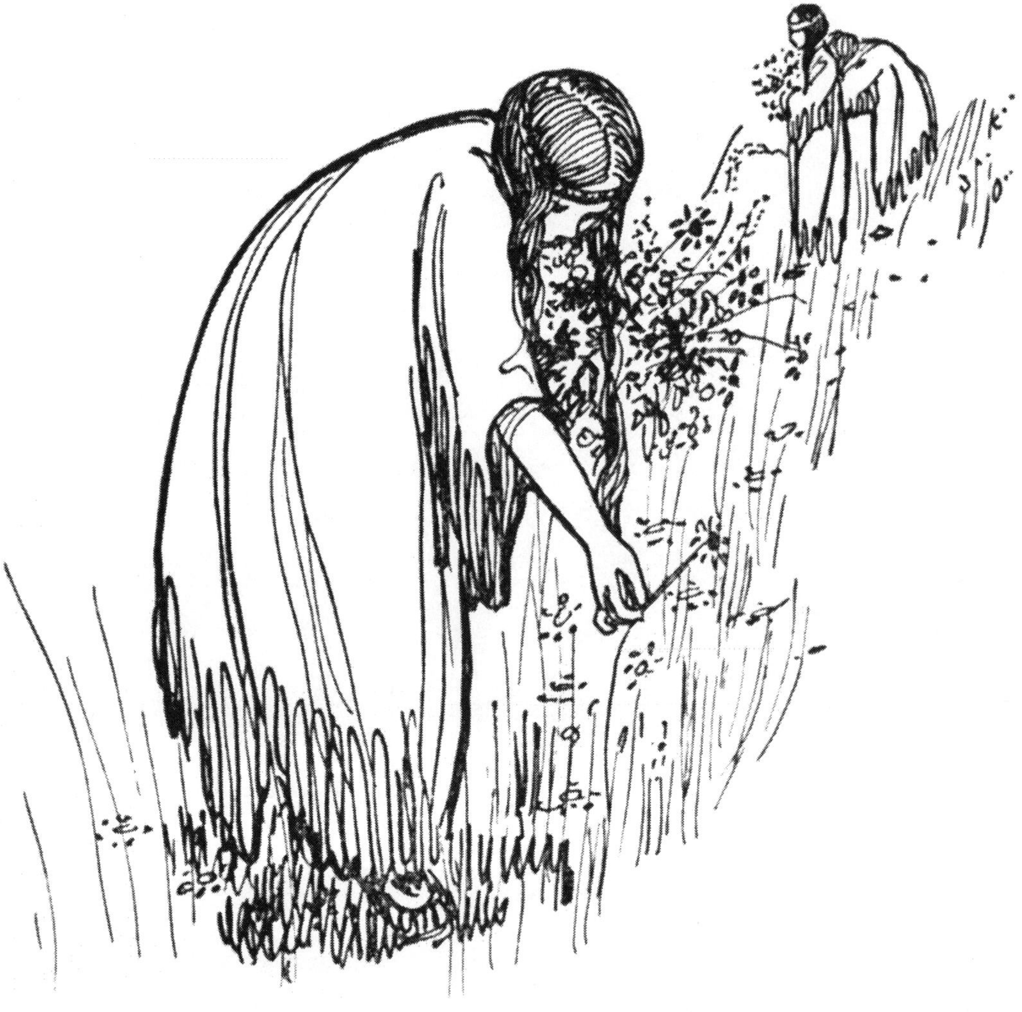

THE LITTLE PARTY SOON SCATTERED TO PICK WILD FLOWERS

By this time the little party had beached the boat on the shore and soon scattered to pick wild flowers.

At the sound of "Wohelo," the girls gathered for their homeward trip.

"My, how my hand and arm burn and itch," exclaimed one of the girls, scratching her arm.

"Oh, perhaps that is plant poison!" cried Soami. "Do you know poison ivy when you see it?"

"No," the girl replied. "What does it look like?"

"My big brother, Ima, explained it this way to me," replied Soami:

Poison Ivy

This vine runs along the ground and climbs trees in just the same way as the beautiful Virginia Creeper. It is quite readily distinguished, however, for Poison Ivy has but three leaves in a cluster, while Virginia Creeper has five leaves.

The poison rash is caused by the irritating juices of the plant.

"My, I wish I'd known that when gathering my flowers," said another girl. "I really believe I've gathered some poison ivy among them. Look, is this the ivy? It has three leaves."

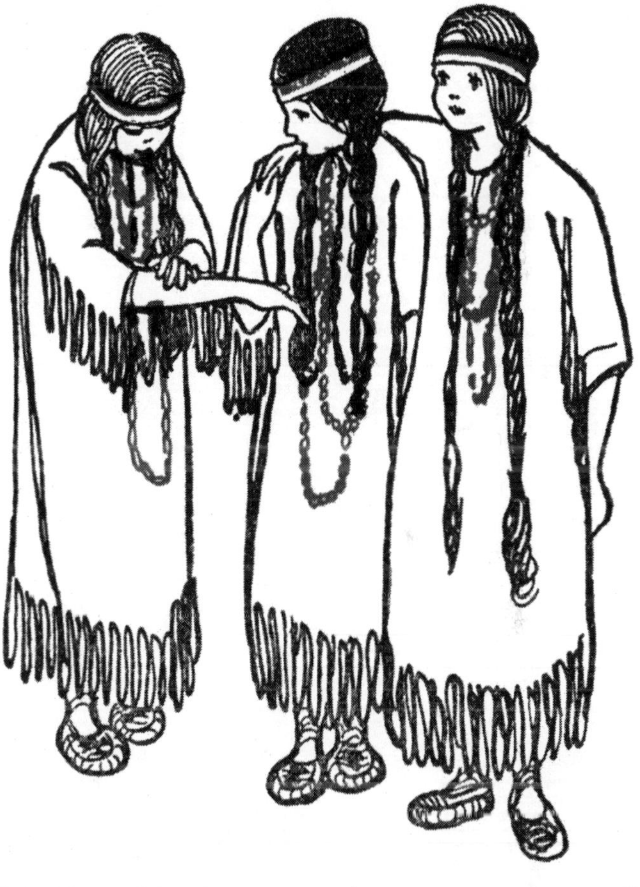

"My, How My Hand and Arm Burn and Itch"

"It certainly is," said Soami. "Please throw it overboard. You may have a case of ivy poison 'for fair,' though not everybody 'takes' poison. Maybe you'll be lucky."

"I sincerely hope so," said the girl so fervently that everybody laughed.

"Well, anyhow, don't scratch!" warned the Guardian of the Fire.

But the next morning's class hour revealed the result of the day's adventures.

Two girls came with bad cases of plant poison, and nearly every girl had been sunburned.

"Well, well," said the assistant nurse, when the girls told of their experiences. "Although I'm sorry for you, this is really very interesting, for it will make you girls see the real helpfulness of our lessons. You can very soon relieve each other of your unpleasant skin irritations, for I shall give you notes on what to do for—

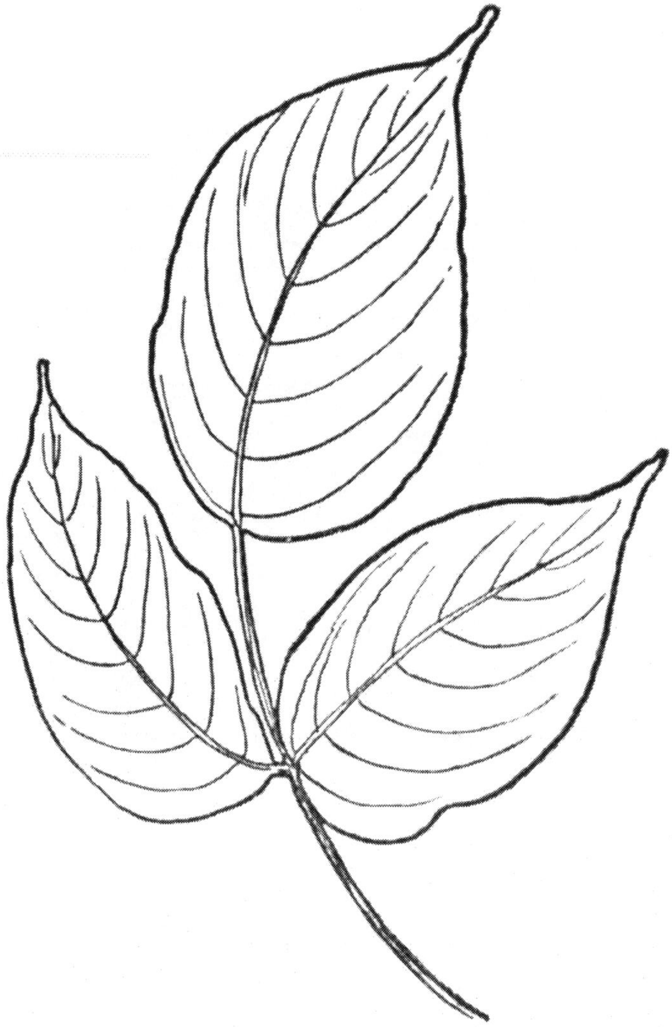

"IT HAS THREE LEAVES"

SUNBURN

(See Reference List)

Sunburn is the result of exposure to the direct or reflected rays of the sun, sometimes causing the skin to blister and peel.

To Prevent:

Before exposure, spread over the face and arms, cold cream or any grease at hand—even cream off milk; or use toilet powder.

Keep the head covered, but have air space between the top of the hat and top of head.

Treatment:

Never wash sunburn.

Never open the blisters.

Mix a lotion of one part limewater to three parts olive oil (sweet oil), and apply.

You see, the treatment is very much the same as for burns.

PLANT POISONING

(See Reference List)

Poison Ivy and a few other plants cause a rash upon the skin after contact with their irritating juices. Everyone should learn to distinguish poison ivy, which has threeleaves, not five, as has the Virginia Creeper (see picture in this chapter). If this poisonous plant were recognized and avoided, there would be but few cases of plant poisoning.

Treatment:

Do not scratch.

Mop on rash a saturated solution of Epsom salt, or boric acid, or baking soda,* with a small "sponge" of absorbent cotton, which is to be thrown away after using. Allow application to dry in the air.

PRICKLY HEAT

Prickly Heat is an itching redness of the skin caused from overheating the body. It appears oftenest on babies; sometimes on older people whose skin is very sensitive.

Treatment:

Bathe with a pure soap, as Castile.

Then bathe with a mixture of one part alcohol to three parts water.

Dust, with talcum powder.

HIVES (NETTLE RASH)

These itching lumps, which resemble mosquito bites, usually indicate stomach or intestinal trouble. They seem to appear after exposure to first, extreme heat; then, to sudden chill. Sometimes they are caused by certain foods; as fish or berries.

Treatment:

For the itching, rub with table salt.

Give a cathartic. Citrate of magnesia is excellent.

Then give a half-teaspoon table salt twice a day for two or three days.

An old-fashioned home remedy is one-quarter teaspoonful cream of tartar in one-quarter glass of water three times a day, at morning, noon and evening, for three days.

If hives persist, see doctor.

"Did you have it all planned to give us this lesson. Miss Helpem?" asked Soami Brave, while the girls bathed their sunburned faces as directed, and treated the poison ivy rash with the Epsom salt solution.

*TO MAKE A SATURATED SOLUTION

*Stir into a small amount of boiled water, all that can be dissolved.

"Do you really want to know?" asked the assistant nurse.

"Please tell us," they begged.

"Well, to tell the truth," replied Miss Helpem, "your needs seemed to require this lesson so much—that I didn't have to invent a game at all—I just put you into practical practice."

"By the way, Miss Helpem," suggested Angie, "would you mind not telling the boys' class about what happened?"

"I promise secrecy," said Miss Helpem. The girls wondered why she and Shesa Brave laughed so heartily—they didn't know that the boys had been given the same promise.

CHAPTER XI

TWO BOYS ARE LATE

TWO boys were absent when the class met for the next lesson.

"How disappointed I am," said Miss Helpem. "This is the first time anyone has missed a lesson."

"Perhaps Tom and Jim will come late," suggested Ibee Brave, and just as he spoke steps were heard.

Ibee opened the door and in came the two boys. Jim was holding a handkerchief to his nose, which was bleeding profusely.

"He didn't want to come in," explained Tom to the nurse, "but I told him you could make it stop. He said he didn't believe so, for he'd tried everything. He kept saying he ought to lie down, and I kept saying he ought to sit up to keep the blood from flowing so easily."

Tom stopped to take a breath. You see he had great confidence in Miss Helpem's first-aid help ever since his experience with his "black eye."

"You were right, Tom," said Miss Helpem, showing Jim to a seat before the class. "If you do not mind, Jim, I will give the boys their lesson now on what to do for—

Nosebleed

(See Reference List)

1. Sit patient upright.
2. Raise arm on bleeding side.
3. Wrap neck and forehead with towels dipped in cold water.

4. Sniff ice water and salt up nostrils. One-half teaspoon salt to a glass of water.

5. Place a piece of ice under the upper lip. Hold ice, wrapped in cloth, on the bridge of the nose.

6. If bleeding still continues, use a small piece of absorbent cotton as a wedge or plug or cork. Fasten a thread to the cotton—to be used to remove it. Dip it into peroxide of hydrogen, and push gently into bleeding nostril with a pencil.

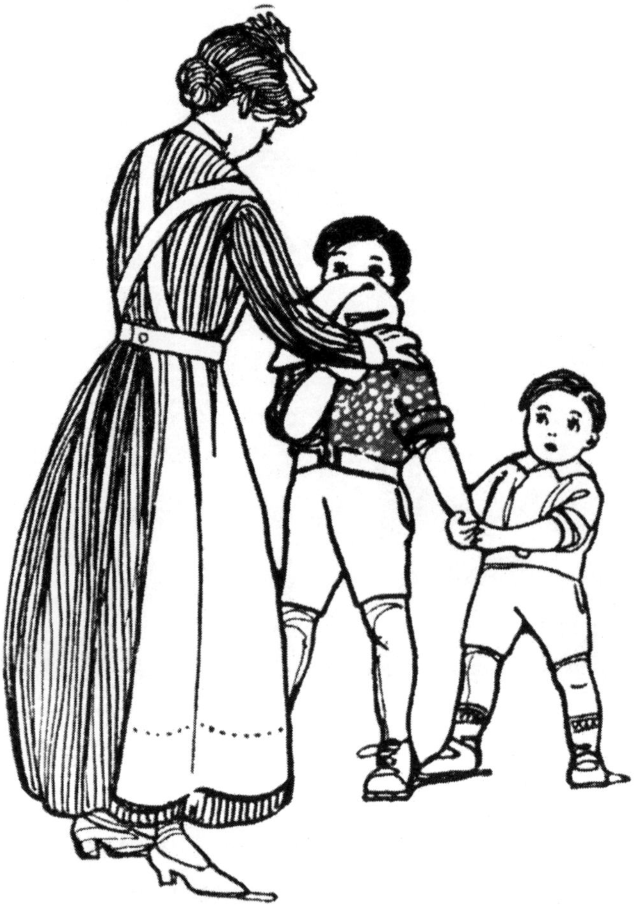

JIM WAS HOLDING A HANDKERCHIEF TO HIS NOSE

Shesa Brave brought the articles needed as Miss Helpem worked, and in a very few seconds after the nurse had used the cotton wedge, Jim's nose stopped bleeding.

It was an excellent lesson for the boys, who didn't realize that the next day they would only be dolls, whose noses may break, but not bleed. Still, if you can remember what to do, those dolls will never mind.

After Jim took his usual place Miss Helpem continued the lesson.

"Let me see," she said, "I think, after nosebleed, perhaps the next most common complaints are earache and toothache and a few other little aches.

"Now, as to—

EARACHE

(See Reference List)

This dreadful pain is generally caused by hardening of the wax in the ear from cold.

To prevent wax from hardening, use a little common *red* (unbleached) vaseline in the ear.

Treatment:

Hold ear over a cloth wrung out of hot water on which is sprinkled some pure alcohol.

With a medicine dropper, drop into ear some warm olive oil; or saturate a small piece of absorbent cotton with the warm olive oil, and place in ear—cover with dry cotton.

(Mothers often use one drop of laudanum in the olive oil, but laudanum is too dreadful a poison for children to handle.)

For watery discharge after earache, it is best to see a doctor, but a sprinkling of boric acid in the ear will usually relieve the trouble.

If earache recurs often, see the doctor.

For Insect in the Ear

Drown insect by filling ear with warm olive oil.

(Mothers sometimes pour a little pure alcohol into the ear to drown and shrink insect.)

For "Something" in the Eye

1. Wink—do not rub.
2. Hold upper lid over under lid, and blow opposite nostril.

eye-cup

An Eye-cup

Remember that almost always an object in the eye will work itself out if the eye is kept closed.

Wash the eye with boric acid solution in an eye-cup.*

Toothache

As soon as possible see a dentist. There would be but little toothache if children were taken in time to a good dentist. This applies even to first teeth, for if first teeth are neglected, the second teeth are affected.

Treatment:

If the tooth feels long, with a throbbing pain, there is trouble with the nerve. Paint gum with iodine, being careful not to swal-

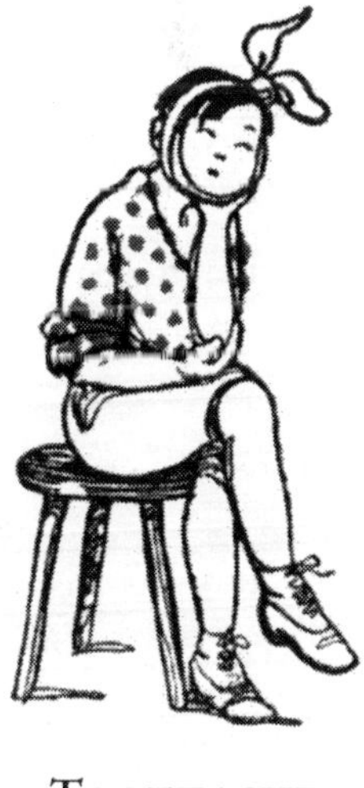

Toothache

*To use an eye-cup, fill it about three-quarters full; hold it over the eye while bending the head forward. Throw head back, holding cup over eye, and open and shut eye several times.

low any. For painting, use a small ball of cotton twisted or tied fast to the end of a toothpick. Never dip the used cotton back into the iodine.

If the tooth aches, look for a cavity, clean out the cavity with a toothpick.

Fill cavity with absorbent cotton wet with essence of peppermint or red pepper water or oil of cloves, and cover with dry cotton.

SPLINTERS

Be careful not to break splinter; pull it out from direction in which it entered.

If no end appears above the skin, open the skin with a needle, *but dip the needle into alcohol first to kill germs.*

Every medicine closet should contain a splinter extractor or tweezers. They cost from five to ten cents.

HICCOUGH

Hiccough is usually caused by indigestion.

Treatment:

A few soda-mint tablets are generally helpful.

Nine or more swallows of water without breathing is a good old-fashioned remedy. So, also, is holding a deep breath.

If hiccough continues, mothers usually give children a cup of warm water in which is dissolved a half teaspoon mustard powder—to cause the child to "throw up" whatever is causing trouble in the stomach.

"Now, I see some of you shuddering," laughed the nurse, "and no one can blame you, but sometimes hiccough becomes very serious, and it is better to take the nasty dose of mustard water than to endanger the heart's action from hiccoughing. But just to console you, I will give some hints as to—

HOW TO STOP NAUSEA (SICK STOMACH)

Cracked ice* held in the mouth, and allowed to melt slowly is excellent.

Soda mint is good.

*An easy way to crack ice is to place a piece about the size of your fist in a strong piece of cloth, and hammer it into bits.

To keep ice chips, lay a piece of wool flannel over a small sieve, and place the chipped ice on this, allowing it to drain into a bowl. Wrap the flannel over the ice. This keeps the warm air out from the ice and the cold air in.

CHILLS

Chills usually show that a person is going to be ill. See a doctor.

Never cool off suddenly. Do not sit down in a cool, breezy place when in a perspiration. It is very dangerous and has caused many a person to "catch his death of cold."

If a person becomes chilled from exposure:

1. Use hot-water bags (or stones or bricks, heated in the oven) or hot stove lids or flatirons, covered with paper or cloth to prevent burning the patient. Place them under the arms and at the feet.
2. Rub the patient's limbs toward the body.
3. Give hot coffee or tea or hot lemonade.
4. Keep well wrapped.
5. Give a hot foot bath in which is a teaspoonful powdered mustard.
6. Wrap in blanket and put to bed.

FAINTING

(See Reference List)

Fainting is caused when too small an amount of blood flows to the head.

To Prevent:

Oftentimes, bending the head forward until between the knees, spreading knees apart, prevents a person from fainting, for the blood then flows to the head.

To restore a person who has fainted:

Keep people away. Patient needs air.

Lay patient flat on floor with no pillow, having fresh air in room. Fan patient.

Loosen clothing about neck.

Hold household ammonia or smelling salts to nose.

Dash a little cold water in face.

Coffee may be given after patient recovers consciousness.

"That is all the lesson for to-day," said the assistant nurse, "and you've all been so attentive that I would like to give you a reward."

"I don't think that we need any reward, Miss Helpem," said Tom Holden, "when you've done so much for us all, already. Gee, you make me feel like being a doctor when I grow up!"

"I hope not all of you feel that way," laughed Miss Helpem. "A doctor in a town full of doctors would have a difficult time making a living."

"That's not true of first-aiders though," said Tom.

CHAPTER XII

PLANS

NO firecrackers, and no toy pistols!" exclaimed Ibee Brave to his Sister Soami, when she told him about the lesson given the girls' class the day before. "That's all right for girls, but I can't imagine boys on the glorious Fourth without firecrackers and pistols!"

"You wait until you hear what Miss Helpem told us. Your lesson comes this afternoon, doesn't it? You may change your mind," prophesied Soami.

"Pooh!" exclaimed Ibee. "I bet I don't! What kind of a fellow would I be, with a brother off with the troops in Mexico, if I were afraid of a toy pistol!"

"Oh, dear me," laughed Soami, "you don't understand. It's not the pistol you ought to be afraid of; it's——"

"Oh, say, talk sense, can't you?" exclaimed Ibee. "What are you driving at, anyhow?"

"That's all for the present, class," replied Soami, tantalizingly, as she ran off with Angie, who had just appeared.

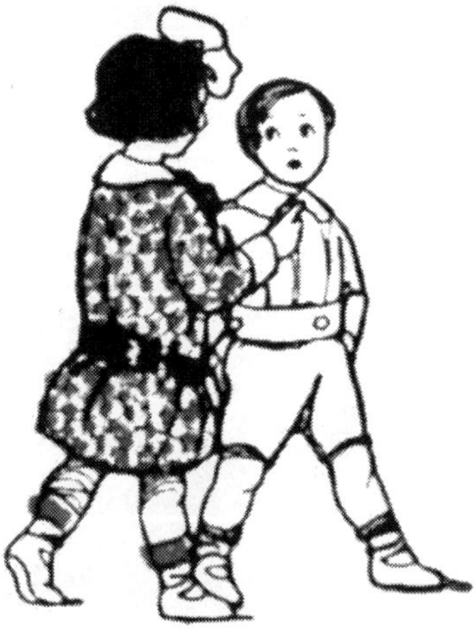

"NO FIRE CRACKERS AND NO TOY PISTOLS!"

Ibee decided to hunt up Tom Holden before going

to class, to find out what he knew. But Tom hadn't heard anything about the question.

"I don't see any harm in a few proper celebrations," said Tom. "What's Miss Helpem's idea, I wonder?"

By the time the class assembled all the boys had heard something about "Miss Helpem's Fourth of July idea," and there was an unusual air of expectancy as the assistant nurse came into the class room carrying—what do you think?—a toy pistol, a bunch of tiny firecrackers, a bunch of medium-sized firecrackers, and some "giant cannon" crackers. Of course, they were very tiny, just the right size for Mary Frances' dolls. The "cannon" crackers were like the tiniest real ones you ever saw.

Miss Helpem had just laid them all on the little glass table near the little glass medicine closet, when Shesa Brave came in carrying a little cannon—which would really "go off, if loaded."

The boys certainly were surprised, for they thought they were to hear these very toys condemned.

"Good afternoon, boys," smiled Miss Helpem, straightening her cap. "This is to be a very interesting lesson. It's our Fourth of July lesson, even though the Fourth doesn't come until next Tuesday. I hope we are all going to have a grand time on the Fourth. The girls' class have planned their part in the town event. Doctor Surecure is in charge, you know. He is planning a civic and patriotic celebration. I shall ask Miss Shesa to read you the program. You will notice that your space is left blank. That is, left open so that we may fill it in to-day. Now, Shesa, read if you please."

Shesa read the—

PROGRAM FOR FOURTH OF JULY CELEBRATION

10.00 A. M. Bugle Call to Village Green.
10.05 A. M. Music by Town Band.
10.10 A. M. Reading of Declaration of Independence.
By the Mayor.

10.20 A. M. Flag Raising. Singing: "Star Spangled Banner."

10.30 A. M. Parade Assembles.

11.00 A. M. Parade Moves:

1. Up Main Street.
2. Through River Avenue.
3. Along Lake Drive.
4. Down Main Street to Village Green.

Order of Parade:

1. Master of Ceremonies on Horseback.
2. Town Council on Horseback.
3. Hearus Band.
4. The Red, White and Blue.

   Borne by Six Boy Scouts.
5. The Boy Scouts.

   (Who will arrange their own program.)
6. Float:

   Camp Fire Girls.
7. The Spirit of '76.
8. Float:

   Our Veterans.
9. Float:

   The Spirit of 1916.
10. Floats:

    First Aiders:

    (*a*) Girls.

    (*b*) Boys.
11. Future Citizens:

    Baby Parade.
12. Float:

    Our Hope.

    School House, over which the Dove of Peace hovers with outstretched wings, just under the American Flag.

Decorated Dollsmobiles.

(Best to be awarded a silver cup.)

Intermission.

2.00 P. M. Bugle Call to Village Green.
2.05 P. M. Music by Hearus Band.
Reading of Lincoln's Address at Gettysburg.
By the Mayor.
2.15 P. M. (*a*) Work Horse Parade.
(*b*) Pony Parade.
3.00 P. M. Prizes Awarded.
3.15 P. M. Singing—"America."
3.30 P. M. Races:
1. Sack Race.
2. Three-legged Race.
(By girls and boys.)
3. Hurdle Race.
4. Fencing Contest.
(Between two boys.)
5. Flag Drill.
By Boy Scouts
and
Blue Birds.
4.30 P. M. Music—Hearus Band.
5.00 P. M. Regatta on Looking Glass Lake.

In the evening, fireworks will be set off on the Village Green in front of Town Hall. Music by Hearus Band.

Notice to the Public.

It will be unlawful to use firecrackers and toy pistols or blank cartridges.

By order of the Town Council.

SIGNED BY THE MAYOR.

"Some program!" commented Tom Holden.

"But why not let us have firecrackers and toy pistols?" asked Ibee Brave.

"Yes, Miss Helpem, why not?" asked half a dozen voices.

"I am prepared for that question," smiled the assistant nurse. "If you will kindly open your note-books, I think by the end of this lesson you will understand that it is not because anyone wishes to deny you fun that you are asked not to use these little toys," pointing to the table, "but because—well, after you have heard the lesson, I think you will know something about the danger from—

GUNPOWDER WOUNDS

Gunpowder is not antiseptically clean. It is very dirty because it contains so many of the deadly germs of lockjaw.

This germ has such a terrible effect upon the body that if not destroyed in time, it causes the jaws to lock so tightly together that they cannot be forced open. Gradually the patient starves to death and finally dies in terrible convulsions of pain.

Toy pistols, firecrackers, blank cartridges, being loaded with gunpowder are very dangerous playthings, and their use should be discouraged. Any physician or nurse will tell you that the hospitals have many deaths from tetanus (lockjaw) after the Fourth of July.

WHAT TO DO FOR POWDER WOUNDS

See a doctor.

Absolutely every wound of this character *must* be treated with anti-tetanic serum.

If doctor is not seen immediately, paint with iodine and anoint with vaseline; but the doctor *must* be seen.

"We never understood the dangers before, Miss Helpem. Now, what will we have in that parade?" spoke up the scout patrol leader.

"We need decide only about the float of the first-aiders," said Miss Helpem. "Your scout-master will confer with you scouts as to the other part of the program."

"Oh, yes," rejoined the patrol leader; "but, Miss Helpem and Miss Shesa, have you thought out anything for our first-aiders' float?"

"To confess the truth," laughed the nurse, "I think Miss Shesa has no less than twenty ideas. Will you make a few suggestions to the boys?" turning to her.

"Miss Helpem has more ideas in a minute than I have in an hour," began Shesa, "but she thought one of my ideas good. It seemed to me that you boys might fix up an improvised first-aid tent on your float, leaving it on the Village Green after the parade. In case any real accident occurred, Miss Helpem could have at hand everything she needed—for somebody might be foolish enough to get hurt. Then you could really do a little actual service by being at her call."

"It sounds wonderfully important," said the patrol leader.

"Only I do wish you boys had had some lessons in bandaging," commented Miss Helpem. "But we'll all do our best, anyway, and look forward with pleasure to those lessons."

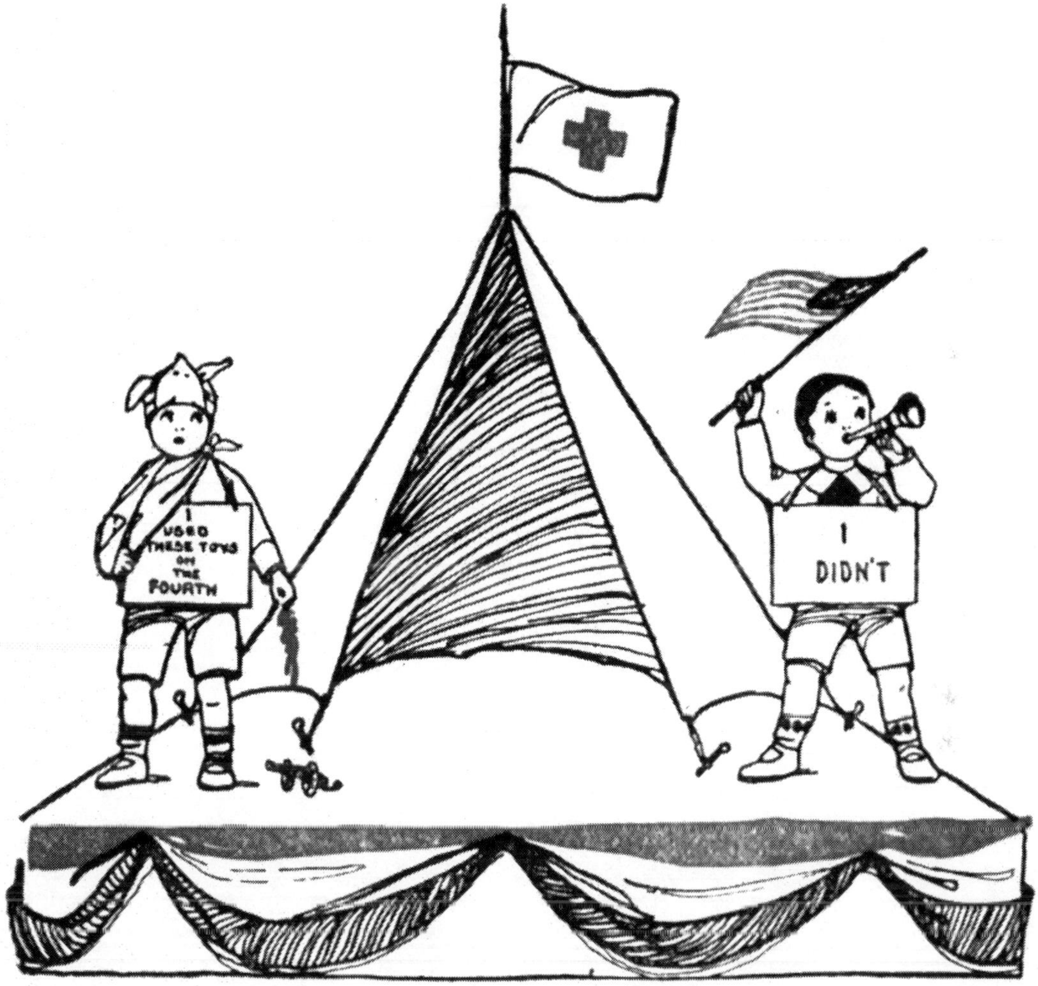

"THAT'S A FINE IDEA"

"Why couldn't we have a little chap all bandaged up, with that toy cannon at his feet and a string of firecrackers and a toy pistol in his hands, with a printed card on him saying, 'I used these toys on the Fourth,' and another little perfectly well chap all dressed in bunting, carrying a flag and holding a horn, bearing a sign, 'I didn't'?" asked the patrol leader.

"That's a fine idea," said Ibee Brave, "but where do *we* come in?"

"We? Oh, we—" the patrol leader answered so lamely that everybody laughed.

"I can tell you, boys, a good way to be better prepared for important work," said Miss Helpem. "If you are willing to take two more lessons before the Fourth, I feel quite certain Miss Shesa will show you the simplest first-aid bandages. She has been taking a full course in first-aid at the hospital, you know. Then, on the float, you may adjust bandages to each other."

"That's awfully kind of Miss Shesa," said the leader. "Will all you fellows come?"

Everybody said yes, and the class was dismissed.

"Say, I wonder what the girls are going to do," exclaimed Tom Holden suddenly on the way home.

"That's so! I wonder why we didn't ask?" said another boy.

"I'll try to find out," said Ibee Brave.

CHAPTER XIII

A SANE FOURTH OF JULY

SOAMI, what are the girls going to do in the parade—on your float, I mean?" asked Ibee, yawning sleepily, as he stretched out in a steamer chair near the hammock in which Soami rocked on the porch of the Brave family's cottage.

"Just—as—though—I'd—tell—you," yawned Soami in imitation of Ibee's manner.

"Say, go on, tell me, won't you?" said Ibee. "I'll tell you a little about ours if you do."

"Yum, yum," sang Soami. "I might possibly tell you a little—you tell first."

"Has Shesa anything to do with your plans?" asked Ibee.

"Oh, so she's going to give you lessons in bandaging, too!" exclaimed Soami, realizing the next instant that she had given a secret away, but the "cat was out of the bag."

Then Ibee began to laugh. "Caught you this time, Sister," he teased. "Shesa wouldn't give me a hint."

"Anyhow, I think you were awful!" said Soami. "I'll watch out for you after this."

"Tell me more? Please do," begged Ibee, but Soami had gone indoors where she felt safer.

. . . . . .

Shesa Brave taught the boys and girls so well that within the week they were quite familiar with the use of—

TRIANGULAR BANDAGES

Bandages cut in the form of triangles are the most useful first-aid bandages, for they are very readily adjusted, and may be applied to so many different uses; for instance:

To hold dressings (compresses) in place.

To support broken or fractured parts of the body (sling).

We will have on hand for our uses:

One large triangular bandage, made from a piece of unbleached muslin one yard square.

Cut the muslin across diagonally, as shown in "A."

Two smaller triangular bandages, made by cutting a large triangular bandage across as in "B."

Of course any piece of goods may be used for a bandage, even handkerchiefs or torn clothing; but we are speaking about the best kind of bandages to have ready for use.

NOTE.—For triangular bandage for doll twenty-one inches high, cut a piece of soft muslin or lawn sixteen inches square. Cut across diagonally for one large triangular bandage. To make the small triangular bandage, cut across the remaining triangular piece.

Triangular bandages are used—

1. Unfolded.
2. Folded.

When the triangular bandage is repeatedly folded on itself it becomes the "cravat" bandage.

The triangular bandage, either unfolded or folded, may be used on any part of the body. The smaller triangles are used for the hands and feet and the jaw.

NOTE.—In the ready-made first-aid packets will be found a triangular bandage, on which are printed sketches of the manner in which the bandage is applied.

You may see how these bandages are used by looking at the picture of Rose Mary, Mary Frances' big dolly, which she bandaged so skilfully that all her friends felt certain that she had been taught by fairy teachers.

If you practice putting these kinds of bandages on your dolls perhaps you will

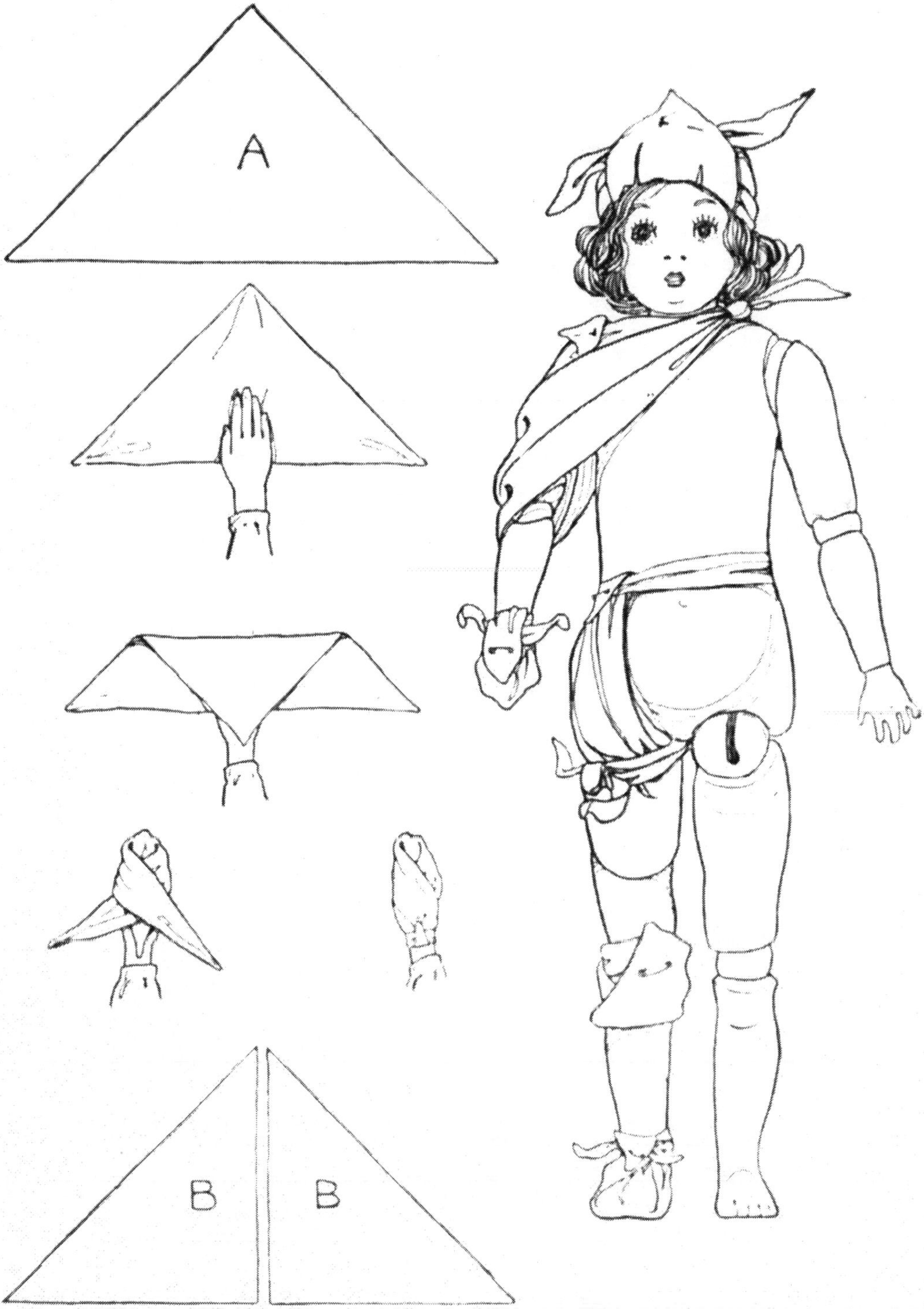

TRIANGULAR BANDAGES

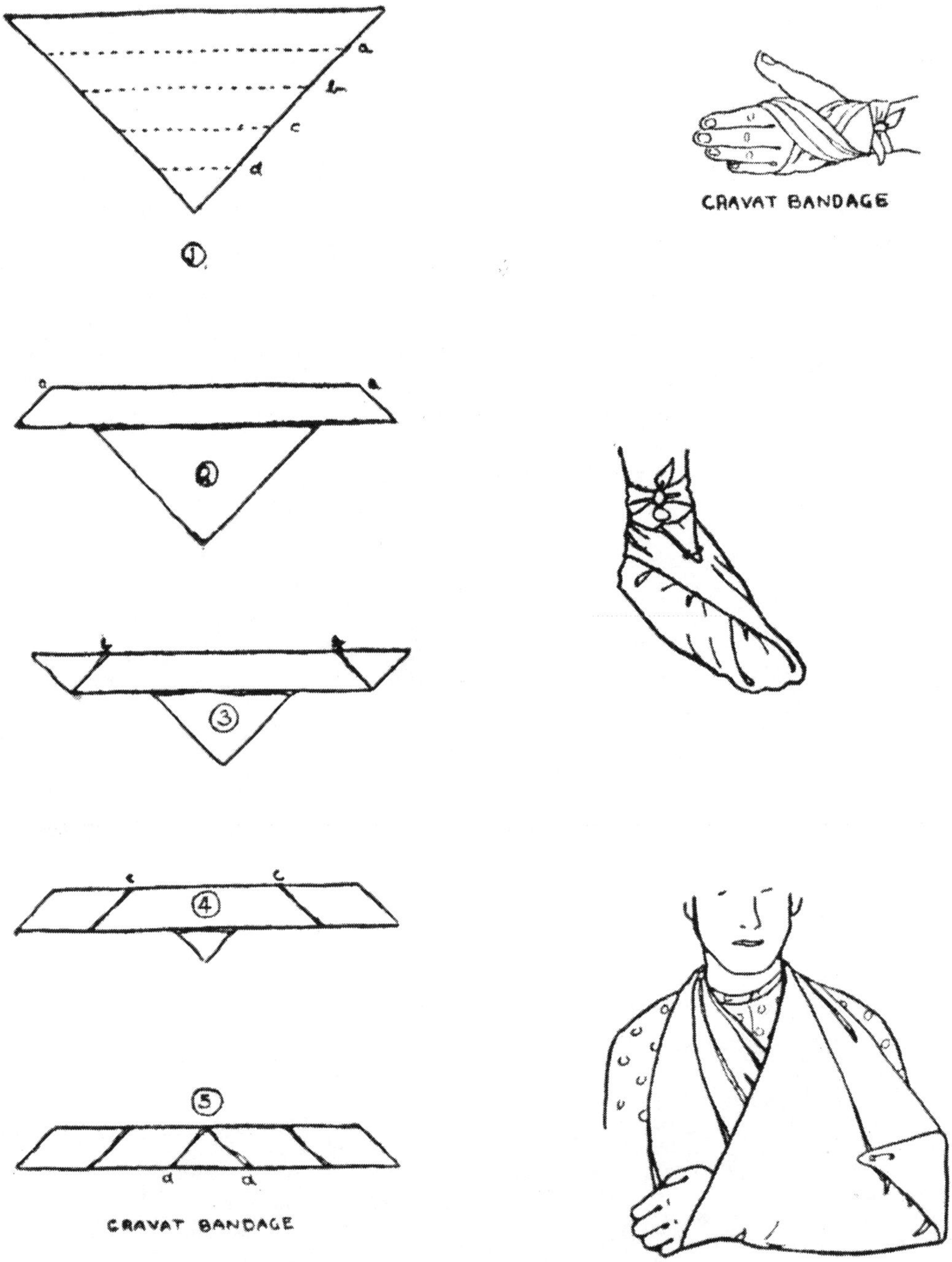

TRIANGULAR BANDAGES

be able some day to help somebody who gets hurt, and seem yourself like a fairy to the person whose pain you helped.

The children became so enthusiastic in practising the various methods of bandaging that it grew to be quite a joke in their homes. Many times they waylaid the various members of their families, whom they wouldn't let go until they were bandaged to look like heroes from the battlefield.

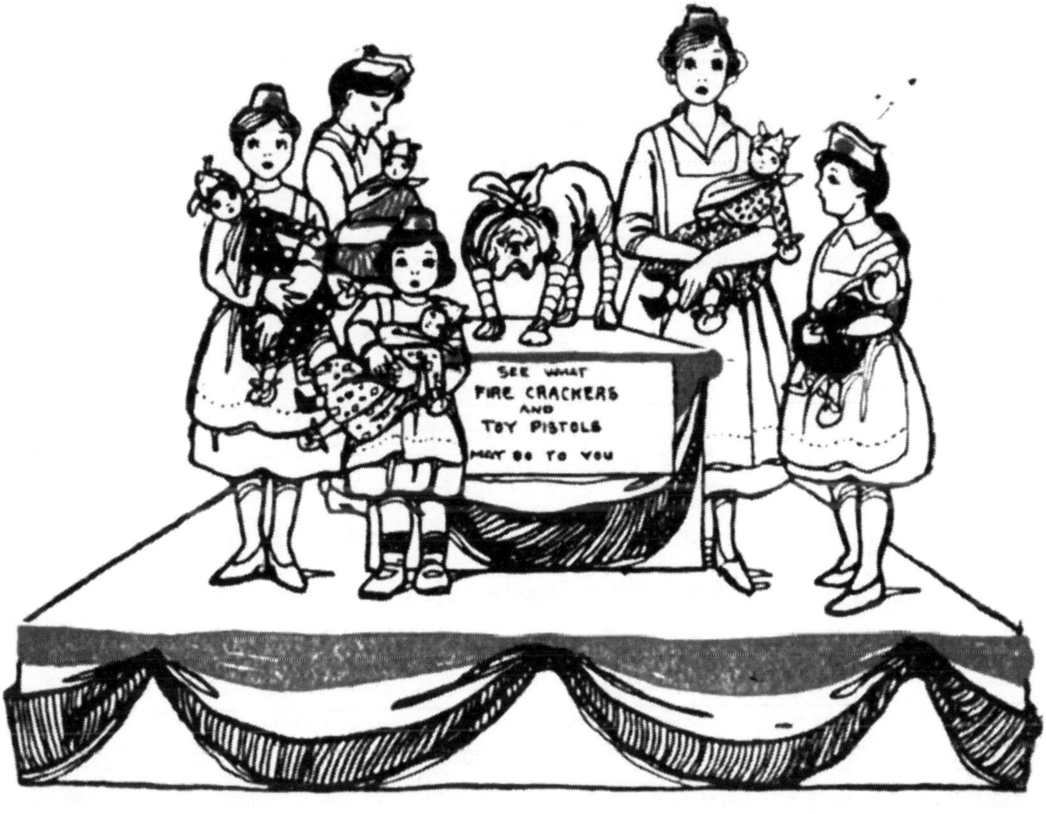

THE GIRLS APPEARED READY FOR THE PARADE

The boys tried in vain to find out what the girls' class had planned for their Fourth of July "float." They taxed their brains guessing, but no one was more surprised than they when the girls appeared ready for the parade, all dressed in nurses' outfits, decorated with a red cross, each carrying a big doll, bandaged, head, hand, arm, foot, in first-aid triangular bandages. In the center of the group, Mike, the Brave family's pet bulldog, was comfortably perched, swathed in bandages. Mike wore a large placard which read:

"See what fire crackers and toy pistols may do to you!"

He seemed to enjoy this particular Fourth, however, more than any other the Brave family could remember.

The boys did have three "real cases" for their first-aid hospital tent.

A very foolish youth, notwithstanding the Mayor's warning, shot off blank cartridges from a revolver, frightening a horse nearby, which broke its halter and ran away, throwing the young man down so hard that he had to be taken to the first-aid tent with a broken arm.

Ibee Brave and Tom Holden happened to be near, and were very proud as they bore the sufferer to the improvised hospital.

They hadn't noticed in their excitement that a little boy had been wounded with the powder from the shot, and felt mortified when two members of the girls' class followed them into the tent with the little patient.

Miss Helpem sent for Doctor Quickenquack, who set the big boy's broken arm and treated the little fellow's powder wounds.

"The worst of it is, young man," said the doctor to the big boy, as he set the arm, "that not all the punishment came to yourself. If these powder wounds become serious for that youngster, you will be blamed."

"I didn't realize, Doctor," replied the young man. "I'll never need any further lesson—after all this, and after I pay my fine."

The other "case" was a lady who fainted when she saw the accident, and was quickly revived in the tent.

"I really believe that this is the best Fourth of July celebration our town has ever known, Doctor," said the Mayor, complimenting Doctor Surecure upon the success of the day. "'A sane Fourth' as you said, will give more pleasure, if people will co-operate, than all the din of firecrackers and thunder of powder. I'm sure we owe you and your able first-aid classes our vote of thanks."

"Miss Helpem deserves all the credit for the first-aid help," replied the doctor.

"Indeed no, thank you, Doctor," laughed Mary Frances Helpem, coming up at that moment. "To the boys and girls of the classes belongs that praise."

CHAPTER XIV

SHESA, A RED CROSS NURSE

"WHAT do you hear from your brother, Shesa?" asked Miss Bossem of Shesa Brave a few days later, as she was leaving the advanced class in first-aid.

The young girl looked troubled. "We haven't heard a word for nearly five weeks," she replied. "I have been thinking seriously of going to the front as a volunteer nurse, hoping I may be able to get news of Ima."

"That seems like an excellent idea to me," said the head nurse. "You, being a member of the American Red Cross Society, can manage very nicely, I think."

So, within a week, Shesa Brave started for Mexico.

She was put on duty in an emergency hospital along the frontier. As the soldiers were brought in she scanned each face eagerly, but many a weary day passed before she had any tidings of Ima.

To every inquiry she sent out, the report came back, "Missing."

A great fear came upon her that Ima had been killed. She couldn't bear the thought that her big handsome brave brother had died without even a record of what had happened; but she worked industriously, nursing other people's brothers and writing letters to the loved ones at home to relieve their anxiety.

While taking a walk one day in her hours off duty, Shesa wandered farther away from the hospital than usual. She was thinking of Ima. Before realizing it, she had lost her direction and found herself in a lovely little valley. The scenery along the border had been so uninteresting, with low cactus plants growing out of the sand, and scrub bushes stretching away in low irregular outline, that this spot came as a delightful surprise.

Spying a little cabin on the side of the mountain above the valley, she decided to inquire the way back, and, quickening her steps, reached it in a short time.

A slovenly woman appeared at the door. Five small children surrounded her, pulling at her skirts as they saw the stranger. The youngest set up a howl of disapproval as Shesa came nearer. In her arms the woman held a baby and in one hand a tin pan of maize or corn. A few chickens came scurrying around the corner of the house as the woman tapped a wooden paddle on the edge of the pan.

The woman stopped and eyed Shesa suspiciously as she came still nearer.

"Good afternoon," said Shesa with a smile. "Do you speak English?"

"Howdy," grunted the woman. "Yes. Hush up, will ye?" to the children, whose noises made conversation difficult.

"United States?" she asked as she looked Shesa's uniform over.

"Yes, yes," replied Shesa. "I'm a nurse."

"Nuss?" said the woman. "Then ye'll know what be ailing him. Come in."

Shesa hesitated a moment before entering the low cabin which was scarcely more than a hut; but, being a brave girl, she thought, "If I am needed, I mustn't hesitate. I'll try to find out what's wanted."

"Tell me about your trouble," she said kindly to the woman. "Is your husband ill?"

"Nope," the woman shook her head, "he be all right. It's a U. S. man we found up yonder," pointing up the mountain road. "Been shot in arm. My man brought him home, but his arm gets worse all time. You know what to do?"

"I think I can help," said Shesa, wishing with all her heart she had brought her emergency kit with her. "Let me see your patient."

The woman led the way into the only bedroom in the cabin. On a rude wooden bed lay a young man, dressed in a much soiled khaki uniform. At the sound of Shesa's voice, he started up. "Sister!" he exclaimed. "Why, this seems too good to be true! Oh, perhaps I'm dreaming. My arm pains so I guess I'm just 'seeing things' from fever."

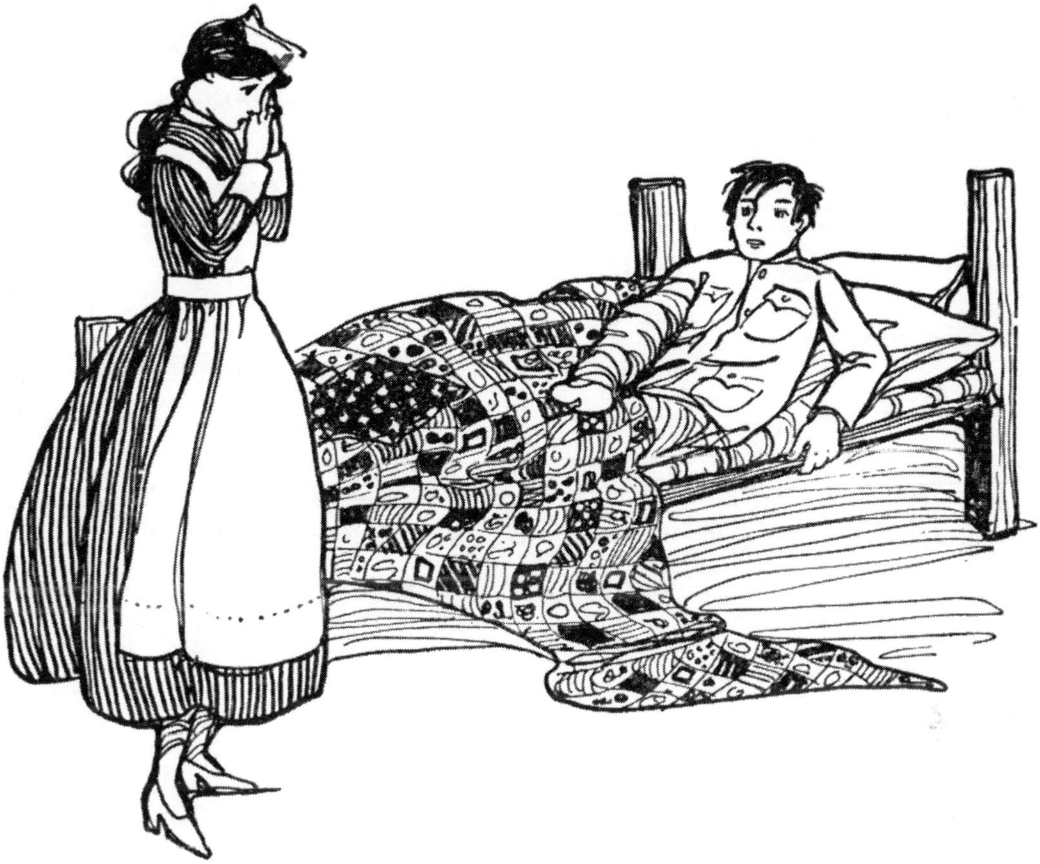

"Sister!" He Exclaimed

For one moment Shesa lost her self-control. Tears filled her eyes and she longed to throw her arms about Ima's neck and cry to her heart's content. "But I must not," she chided herself. "I must do everything I can to help him."

"It's not a dream, Ima, dear," she said as naturally as if they were in their far-away home. "You are ill and certainly do need me. Let me see your arm."

The sight of his poor wounded arm made her feel sick, for it evidently had been neglected from the first.

"How did it happen?" Shesa asked, as she tore her apron into bandages and directed the woman to boil some water on the open fire which she had seen outside.

She saw that Ima wanted to talk, sick and weary as he was.

"I was taking a stroll alone one evening," he explained, "not thinking of the least danger, for our camp lights were scarcely out of sight. Suddenly I heard the report of a gun, and felt an awful pain in my right arm. One of the bandits had evidently spotted me from ambush. I'd have been all right, but the fellow or an accomplice sprang upon me, and after a struggle knocked me senseless and took my emergency kit and everything else useful away from me. The settler who owns this cabin found me and brought me up here on his shoulders. His wife did what she could for my wound, but it became infected almost immediately, and I was too weak from loss of blood to walk back to camp, even with the man's help. Besides, in some way, I had a sprained ankle."

"Well, dear, you are going to be helped in every way soon, so don't talk any more," said Shesa, taking off some of the dirty rags which the woman had tied clumsily upon Ima's ankle. She bathed the ankle in hot water and bound it firmly in a figure-of-eight bandage, which gave him the first ease from pain since the accident.

She replaced the outside layers of the dirty bandages on his wounded arm. "The wounds may bleed if I take the dressings off," she decided wisely, "and I have no remedies here."

"I wonder why the man didn't go for help?" she thought.

Just at that moment Ima whispered, "I would have sent word to camp, but for some reason the settler seems afraid—of the bandits, maybe."

"Well," said Shesa, "you rest here, and we'll soon have help."

"But, Shesa, it will be dangerous for you to go," said Ima. Then suddenly, "Why, how did you happen to come here, anyhow?"

"Never mind, dear, I'll explain all that later," replied Shesa.

"But I want to hear now," insisted Ima, his eyes bright with fever. So to satisfy him, Shesa briefly related the story of her little walk.

"Now," she added "since the emergency hospital is so near, you need not worry until I come back?"

He promised to try not to worry, and fell into a dozy sleep within a few minutes.

CHAPTER XV

A TELEGRAM FROM MEXICO

SHESA hurried along by the path she thought she had taken to reach the cabin, but after walking ten minutes, found herself going in the wrong direction.

"How dreadful!" she exclaimed, "when I am in such a hurry!"

She looked about her. "It is nearing sunset," she whispered, looking at the sky. "Oh, I wish I knew the way!"

Just at that moment a noise in the underbrush startled her. Although very brave, she was dreadfully afraid of snakes, even harmless ones, but she laughed when she saw a tiny prairie dog scamper out of the bushes, stand on his hind feet and look about him with blinking eyes.

"How foolish I am!" she thought, but shuddered again as she heard someone stepping up behind her.

"I beg pardon," said a gentlemanly voice—and turning, you can imagine how relieved Shesa was to see a United States soldier standing with his hat in his hand.

"Oh," she cried happily, "I'm so thankful to see you. Will you help me find my way to the emergency hospital?" Then she stopped and laughed. "I must apologize for speaking this way," she said, "but you will understand my excitement when I explain all that has happened to me this afternoon."

The soldier quickly led the way as she talked.

They soon arrived at the emergency hospital, and after Shesa's explanation, the doctors took her in a field ambulance up to the cabin, the soldier showing the way.

Within two hours, Private Brave lay on a clean white cot, with clean dressings on his arm and comforting broth in his stomach.

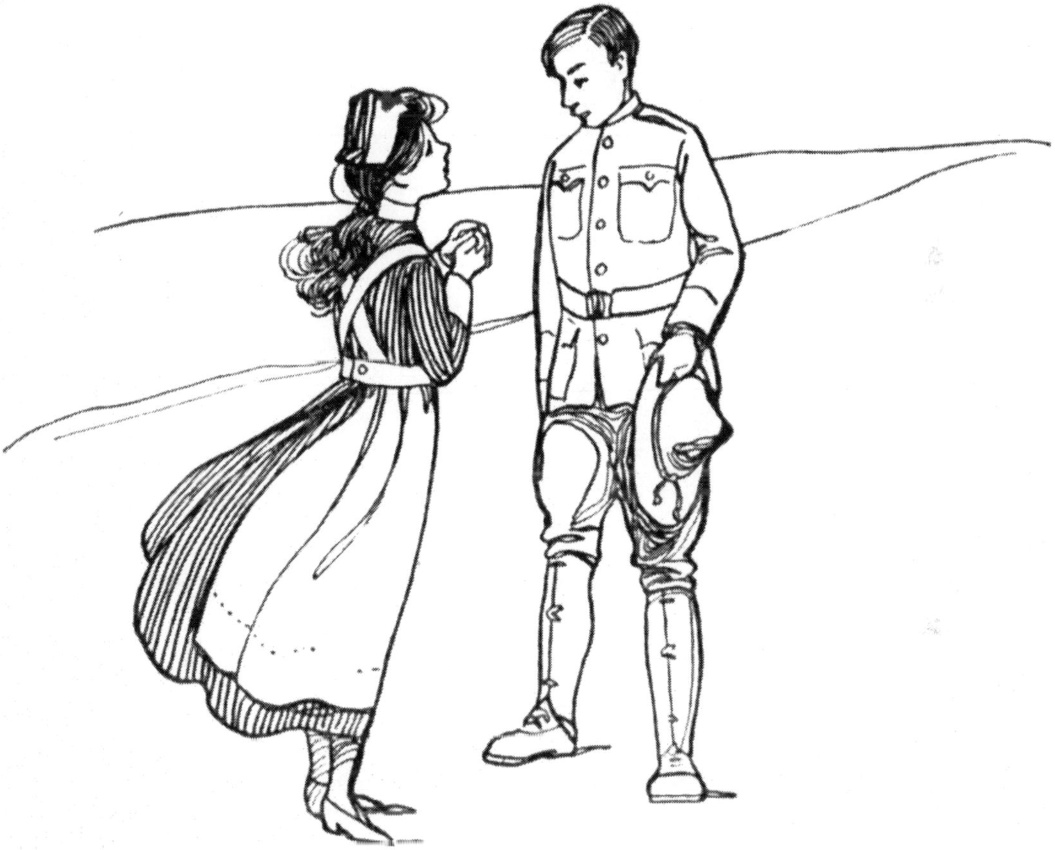

Will You Help Me Find My Way to the Emergency Hospital?"

"I feel a hundred per cent better already," he said to Shesa as she kissed him good-night. "In the morning I'll be well."

But in the morning the doctors shook their heads. "I'm afraid that arm will have to be amputated," said the chief surgeon.

"Oh, Doctor!" exclaimed Shesa, "can't it be saved?"

"If it is saved," said the doctor gruffly, not liking to show how sorry he was for

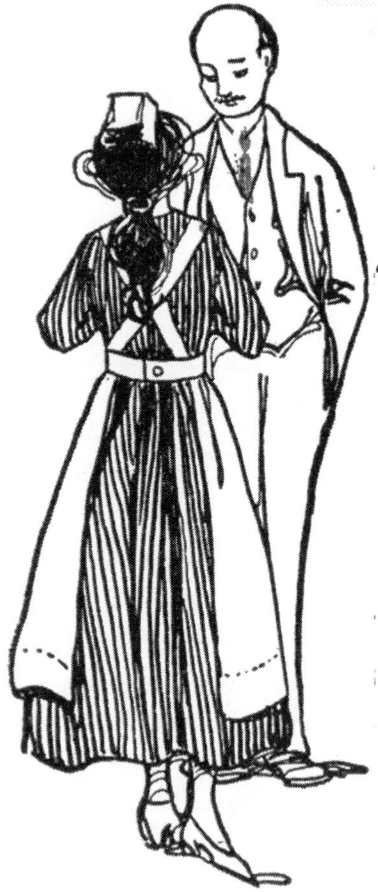

"OH, DOCTOR! CAN'T IT BE SAVED?"

the pretty nurse, "it will be saved for a dead man. A neglected infected wound, even small, may mean gangrene. This is a large, badly neglected infected wound!"

Shesa bit her lips and held back the tears, saying, "Of course, if it's to save his life, Doctor—" Then she went out to telegraph to her family.

The telegram read:

Ima found, wounded. Will bring home soon as possible.

Shesa.

"Oh, how I hope all comes out right," she thought.

. . . .

CHAPTER XVI

PRIVATE BRAVE'S ADVENTURES

THREE weeks later, a soldier with one arm and his very attentive sister were looked upon with much interest by the other passengers on a steamer going to New York.

Ima stood the journey well, but when they arrived at the station, Shesa decided to take himdirect to the Dolls' Hospital to rest instead of home, where he would be under a good deal of excitement.

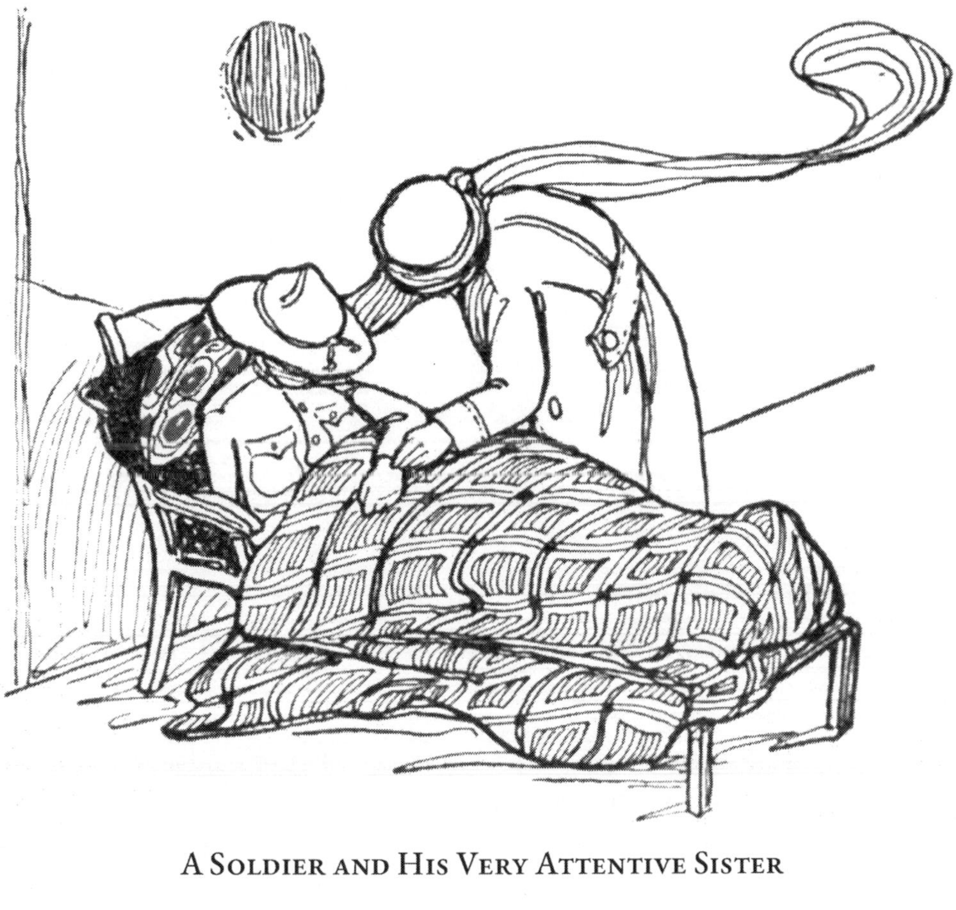

A SOLDIER AND HIS VERY ATTENTIVE SISTER

So it was in the Dolls' Hospital that the Brave family came together again, rejoicing in the escape of their soldier. Even Mike, the dog, was allowed to come, and no one greeted him with more joy than did their family pet.

Private Brave didn't mend as well as the doctors and nurses had hoped. Within a week after his arrival at the hospital, an abscess developed on his left forearm, which caused everyone to worry, and another operation was all that saved poor Private Brave from losing his only remaining arm.

The assistant nurse dressed and bandaged this abscess with—

ROLLER BANDAGES

(See Reference List)

Roller bandages are usually made of long straight pieces of gauze. This material "gives" to the form of the arm much better than muslin. Never put a bandage on wet, for it shrinks and is too tight when dry.

You will be interested in seeing a picture on page 99 of how a roller bandage is applied to an arm or leg.

This picture shows one of Mary Frances' big dolls bandaged in roller bandages.

The two-and-a-half-inch wide roller bandage four or six yards long is the size most used for grown-up people, although narrower ones are needed for fingers.

On the doll's body inch-wide bandages were used, and the ends were sewed in place. To prevent slipping, strips of adhesive plaster were placed over the folds of the edges.

Under the assistant nurse's kind care, Private Brave soon grew better and was able to take an interest in the other patients.

He begged to be allowed to visit the boys' ward, where he wouldn't be so lonely.

There was great excitement among the boys in the ward, none of whom were very ill, when a real soldier came to visit them.

They coaxed him to tell them about his adventures.

They liked best the story about how he lost his arm, and this one about the stolen baby:

THE WAY PRIVATE BRAVE SAVED A BABY'S LIFE

"We were riding along one day, when I thought I heard a baby's cry. None of the other boys seemed to hear it, and as we were not riding in order, I headed my

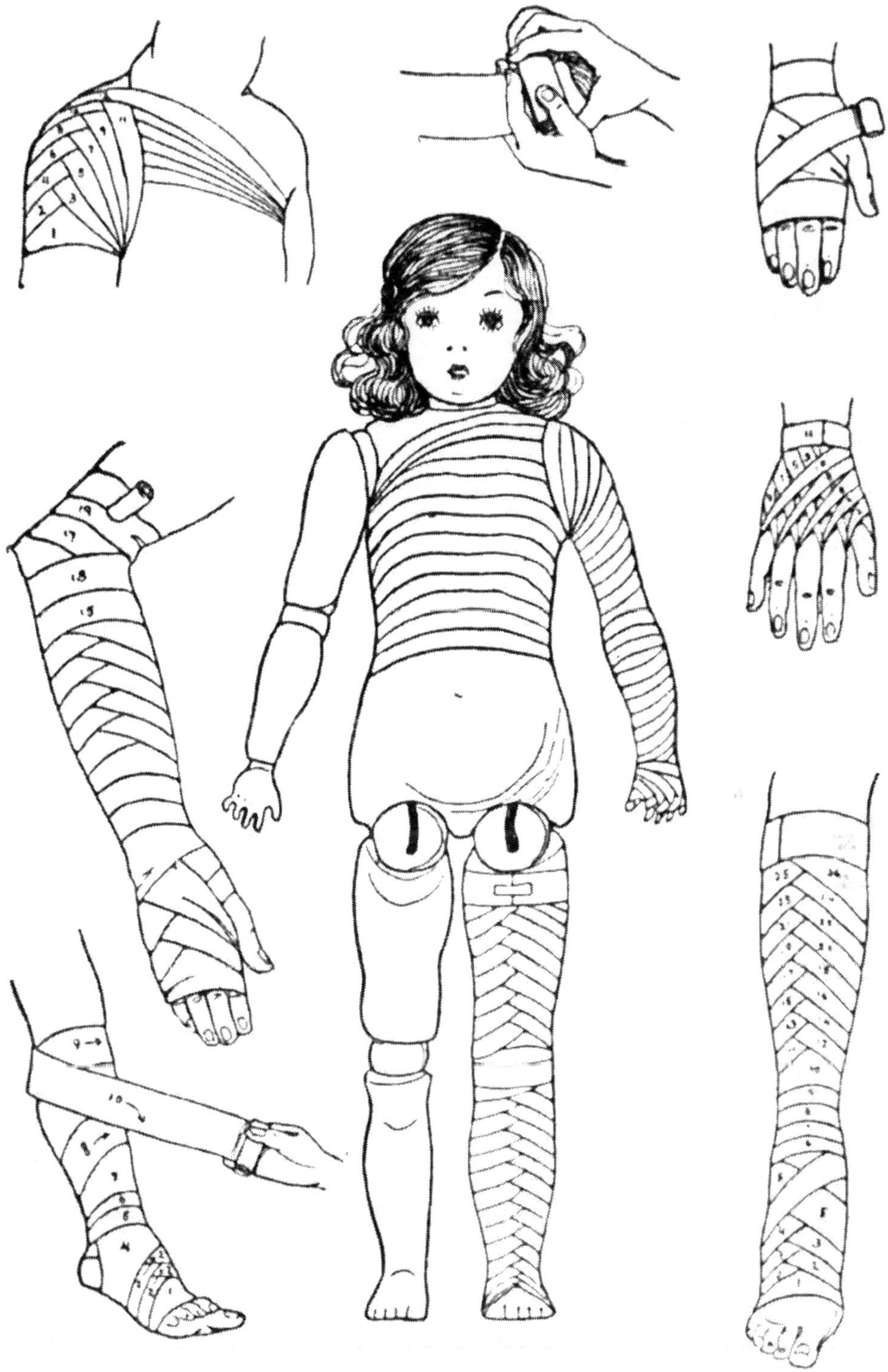

ROLLER BANDAGES

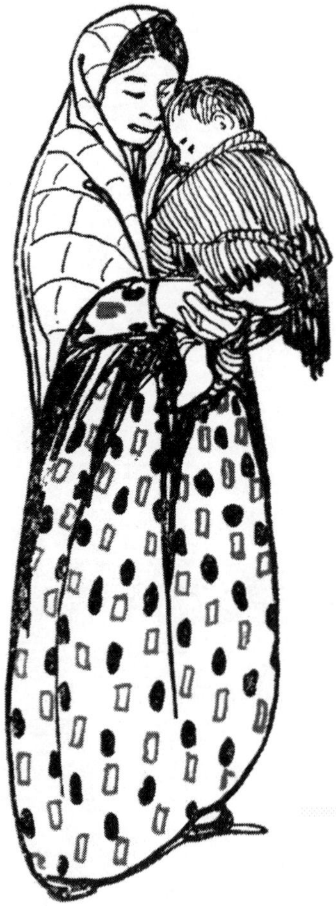

WE PUT THE BABY INTO HER ARMS

horse toward the sound. I had about concluded that I was mistaken, when the horse stopped short. The crying had ceased by this time.

"I looked down, and there among the sage-brush, at the horse's feet, was a little baby about a year old. How it came in such a place, I have no idea. There was no house within forty miles, and we hadn't met a soul.

"I got off my horse and picked the little thing up and rode with it to our captain. It appeared to be half starved and surely could not have survived much longer.

"We carried it with us into camp, fed it and took care of it as best we could.

"On making inquiries, we found the baby had been stolen from some poor white settlers. Who did it or why, no one ever found out.

"When the poor mother came into camp and we put the baby into her arms she was the happiest woman I ever saw."

"Wasn't that grand!" cried Bobby to Sammy, the little lame boy in the next bed. Sammy was the plaster-of-Paris doll Mary Frances had bought for a nickel at the children's fair.

All the patients were sorry—and the doctors and nurses, too—when the time came for Private Brave to leave the hospital.

He had been so bright and cheerful that they would miss him greatly.

He felt sorry, too, in a way, for so many interesting things had happened; for instance—but perhaps you would rather hear the story of the mad dog as Private Brave told it to his family.

CHAPTER XVII

THE MAD DOG

PRIVATE BRAVE was comfortably seated in the home living room with his family gathered around to hear what had happened while he was in the hospital.

"It was about four o'clock in the afternoon," he began. "I had just finished telling the boys about saving the baby, and all my other experiences which you know, when suddenly we heard a woman crying as she rushed past the ward door.

"'Oh, Doctor,' she sobbed, 'will he die—will my little boy die? He didn't know the dog would bite, poor child! He says the dog isn't mad, but everybody else says he is!'

"'Come,' said the doctor, 'mad or not, we'll fix this young man up so he'll be quite safe. I'm glad you brought him to me immediately.'

"I was on my feet in an instant, and ran to the office door, for I was very anxious to hear what would be done for the little boy.

"'This must be cauterized, Nurse,' said the doctor. 'Get nitrate of silver ready.'

"He dipped a wooden stick into the poison and turned it around in the wound, the little boy screaming with the pain.

"'Oh, Doctor,' asked his mother, 'must he be hurt so much?'

"'Safety must first be considered,' replied the doctor. 'We are probably destroying the dreadful germs of hydrophobia. And, next, this little boy must be given Pasteur treatment with the wonderful serum used to prevent hydrophobia, for hydrophobia means the most terrible suffering anybody could imagine. Of course, no one is quite certain that the dog was mad; for many a time a dog which has been nearly crazed with thirst, or been the victim of bad boys' pranks, has been thought mad.'

"'But this doggy wasn't mad,' the boy cried out, forgetting his pain. 'A bad boy was twisting his tail and the poor doggy thought I did it because I was near!'

"'Are you certain, little fellow?' asked the doctor.

"'Yes, sir, and after he bit me, a big man beat him with his cane, and the poor doggy ran yelping down the street. Oh, how you made my arm ache, Doctor!'

"'Poor boy!' said the doctor, 'I really had to hurt you.'

"'What should I have done, Doctor, if we had been miles from a physician?' asked the mother.

"'That's a good question,' replied Doctor Surecure. 'I will tell you the simplest treatment for an untrained person to use—

FOR DOG BITE

(See Reference List)

Whether there is danger of hydrophobia or not, if bite is on limb, tie a cloth tightly around limb between wound and body, and encourage bleeding by squeezing. Wash with soap and hot water. Apply iodine. Loosen cloth in an hour.

If there is the slightest danger of hydrophobia, get patient to a doctor! If impossible to get a doctor, apply nitrate of silver, or pure carbolic acid with a soft stick. But it seems that there are few places where a doctor cannot be consulted within twenty-four hours,—who will see that the patient is given Pasteur treatment to prevent hydrophobia from developing.

"Well, I am certainly glad to learn that, my son," said Private Brave's mother. "We had a terrible fright the day the little boy was bitten, for somebody said that our Mike did it."

"What!" exclaimed Private Brave. "Did anybody dare accuse this most faithful and wonderfully brave dog-member of the Brave family?"

Mike had been lying at his young master's feet; in fact, he hadn't left him since he came home—not even to eat his dinner. On hearing his name, Mike stood up, wagging his tail so hard that you would have thought it would drop off unless it was nailed on.

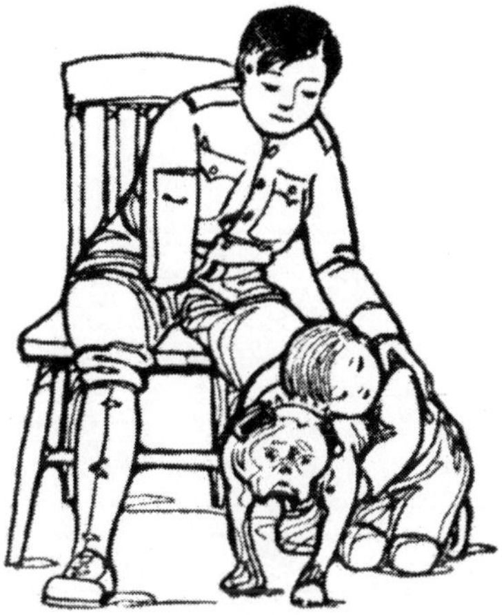

"IT WASN'T YOU, MICHAEL, OLD BOY!"

He looked inquiringly upon the family, his mouth open and his intelligent brown eyes questioning what all this talk meant.

"It wasn't you, Michael, old boy, good old fellow!" exclaimed Ibee, petting him.

"Bow! Bow!" barked Mike, and Ibee declared he smiled.

"Well," said Private Brave, "that was—" He didn't finish the sentence, for at that instant the next door neighbor came running into the room.

"Oh, come, Miss Shesa!" she exclaimed. "My baby's dying—she's swallowed poison."

CHAPTER XVIII

THE POISONED BABY

SHESA hastened away with the neighbor, for she knew that any delay might cost the baby's life. She could hear the little girl's agonizing screams.

"Ibee, run for the doctor," she called.

"We must work until the doctor comes," she said to the distracted mother. She was wise enough to realize that it would be best to keep the mother busy.

"What kind of poison—do you know?" asked Shesa anxiously, as they ran up the steps of the porch.

"Lye," answered the mother briefly. "The maid was scrubbing the kitchen steps, and left the can of lye on the floor. Baby came along, saying 'dink, dink,' and before Sally Ann could get into the door, baby had swallowed a mouthful. It couldn't have been very strong, for Sally Ann had filled up the can with water."

Shesa took the baby on her lap and looked into its poor little burnt mouth.

"Bring a glass of water and some vinegar," she ordered. When they came, she diluted the vinegar with water giving the baby a teaspoonful at a time.

"Bring the juice of a lemon," she said. This she diluted, giving it to the baby in the same way.

It must have stopped some of the suffering, for the little one began to seem more comfortable.

"Now, the beaten white of an egg in water," she said at length. Of this she gave the baby a tablespoonful; then a tablespoonful of olive oil, holding its little mouth shut to make it swallow.

By the time the doctor arrived, the baby had fallen asleep on Shesa's lap.

"You have saved this baby's life, Miss Brave," said the doctor. "If it hadn't been for prompt action, the child might have died."

"People are so careless with poisons," he went on. "Poisons should never be placed within the reach of little children. All bottles should be labeled plainly, and the stoppers should be tied about with a piece of gauze—not very attractive, I admit, but one of the best safeguards against making a mistake as to the 'right bottle.' Poisons should not be kept in the general medicine closet, but in a place by themselves—unless we except iodine, which has such a decided odor that it may be kept in a more accessible place, ready for its many uses."

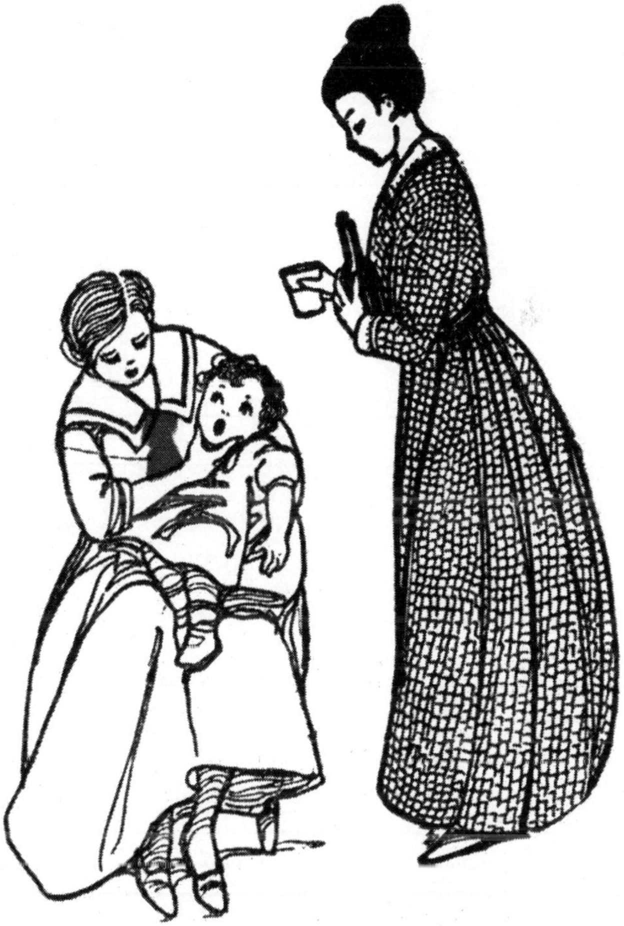
"BRING A GLASS OF WATER AND SOME VINEGAR"

After complimenting Shesa again on her treatment of the baby, and leaving some medicines for both the baby and the baby's mother, the doctor went away.

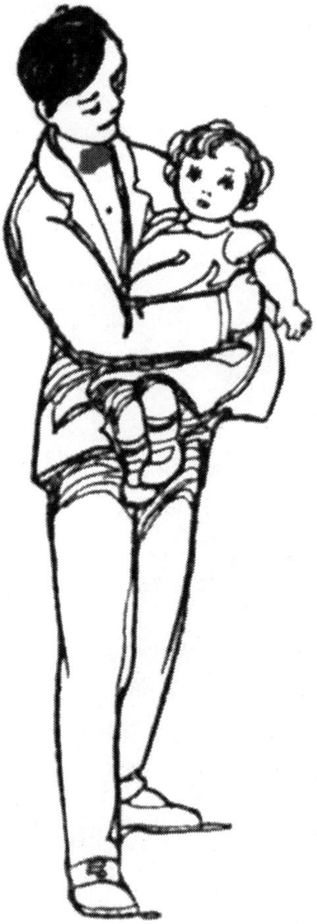

"YOU HAVE SAVED THIS BABY'S LIFE, MISS BRAVE"

Shesa was met by her mother as she started home.

"We are all so anxious, dear," she said, "to learn how the baby is."

"The baby's all right," smiled Shesa.

"How thankful Ima will be!" exclaimed her mother. "It brings tears to my eyes to see how interested that dear boy is in everybody, thinking so little about his own misfortunes. Think of a young man just at his age losing an arm!"

"Father told me that last night when he tried to express a little sympathy, Ima said, 'Well, Father, it is a loss; but you know, I have one arm left!'" Shesa replied.

"Wasn't that wonderful!" exclaimed Mrs. Brave.

"It certainly is wonderful how bravely he takes his troubles," replied Shesa. "Father said he thought that it really required more bravery to feel that way than to go to the battlefield."

By this time they had reached home, and Shesa had to tell everybody about the saving of the life of the poisoned baby.

CHAPTER XIX

HURRAH FOR OUR HERO

THE Brave family were not the only people who admired Private Brave's cheerful acceptance of his fate and his determination to make his left hand learn to do the work of two hands.

One day when he was running the lawn mower over the lawn in front of the house, Doctor Quickenquack stopped in his dollsmobile.

"Hello, how's the 'General'?" he called. "Can't you jump in and take a ride? Hope you're not too busy to have a little holiday."

"Thank you, Doctor," said Private Brave, "it's certainly kind of you to ask me. Will you wait until I put this mower away and get my coat?"

He had to lock the door, for none of the family were home, but he hopped into the car in a minute's time. The doctor started the engine and away they rode toward Painted River and Looking Glass Lake. It was a beautiful morning and Private Brave enjoyed the ride very much.

"If you will just let me out here, I'll walk home from this corner," said he as they came to River Avenue.

"Not much, sir; you're kidnapped," laughed the doctor as he drove on toward the hospital.

"First, your lunch; then a visit to the boys' ward," said the doctor. "That's your program, sir."

Private Brave was delighted with the idea, and how he enjoyed his lunch after the ride!

When he went with the doctor to the boys' ward, you can't imagine how surprised he was to see all his own family. Not only they were there, but also the boys' class and the girls' class in first-aid.

Besides these, wore Miss Bossem and Miss Helpem and Doctor Surecure and even the ambulance driver, Billy.

Doctor Quickenquack led Private Brave under an American flag which was draped in one corner of the room.

"Dear Private Brave," said Doctor Surecure, clearing his throat, "it is my pleasure to present to you a gift from some of your many admiring friends."

Private Brave blushed at the praise, and smiled as Miss Helpem carried forward a box which she placed on the little table beside him.

He opened the lid and lifted out a beautiful little hand-embroidered silk flag.

"Perhaps we'd better help you open the box the rest of the way," suggested Doctor Surecure. "Let us step into the next room."

When the doctors and Private Brave came back—what do you think? Private Brave was waving the beautiful little silk flag in the hand of a new wooden arm, so skilfully made that it had almost human action.

"Hurrah!" shouted the boys and girls in delight. "Hurrah! Hurrah for Private Brave! Hurrah for Our Hero!"

"Hurrah! Hurrah!" they shouted together at the top of their lungs.

"Hurrah for Private Brave! He's—

Prepared for less,
  Prepared for more,
Prepared for peace,
  Prepared for war!

Prepared for well,
  Prepared for ill,
Prepared to save
  The doctor's bill!

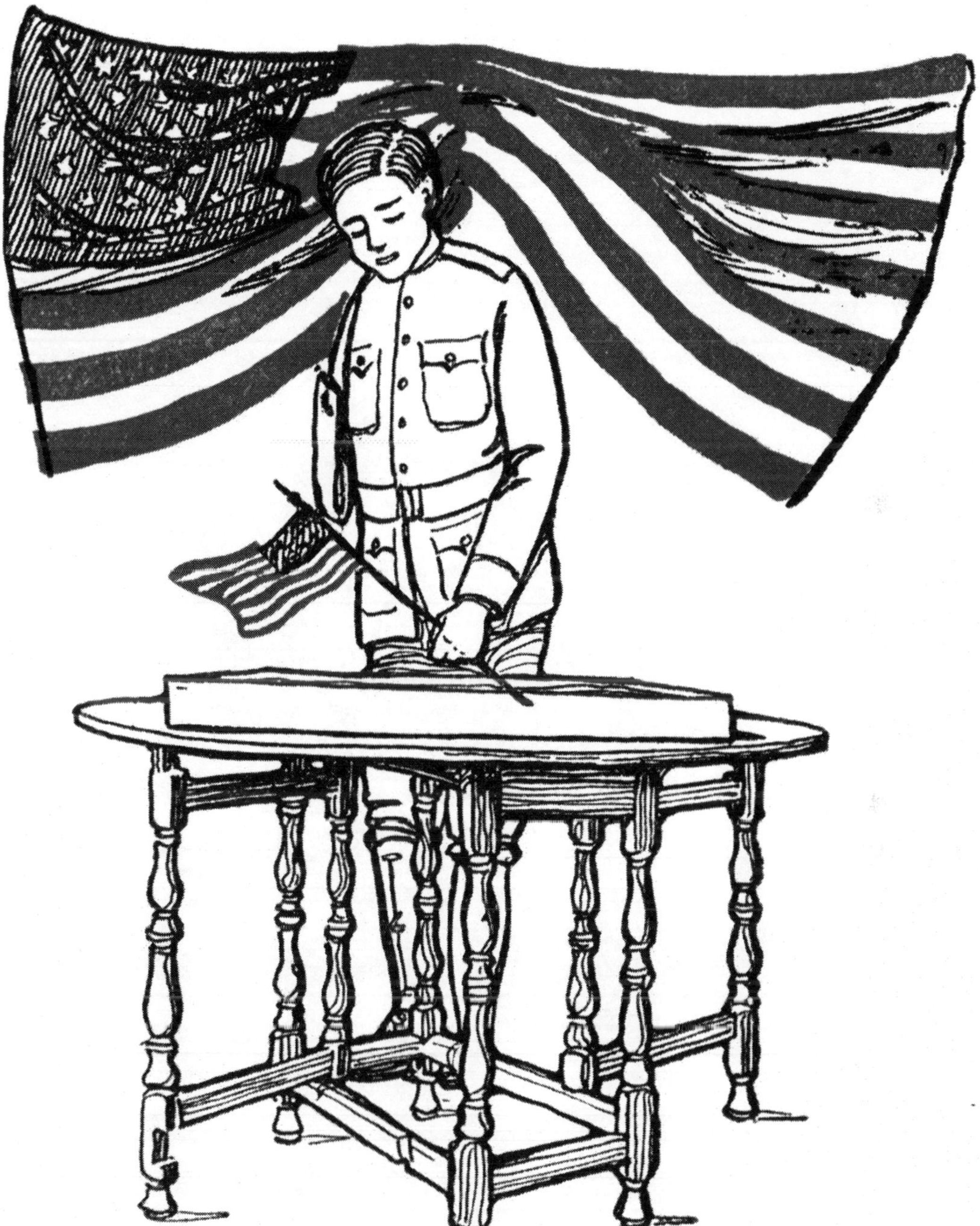

He Opened the Lid and Lifted Out a Beautiful Little
Hand-Embroidered Silk Flag

Prepared for calm,
Prepared for strife,
Prepared for anything
In life!

. . . . . .

"Oh, Billy," cried Mary Frances, after it was all over, "I'm so thankful to you for your birthday present."

"What do you mean?" yawned Billy.

"Why, for the day we've just spent together in the playroom," said Mary Frances.

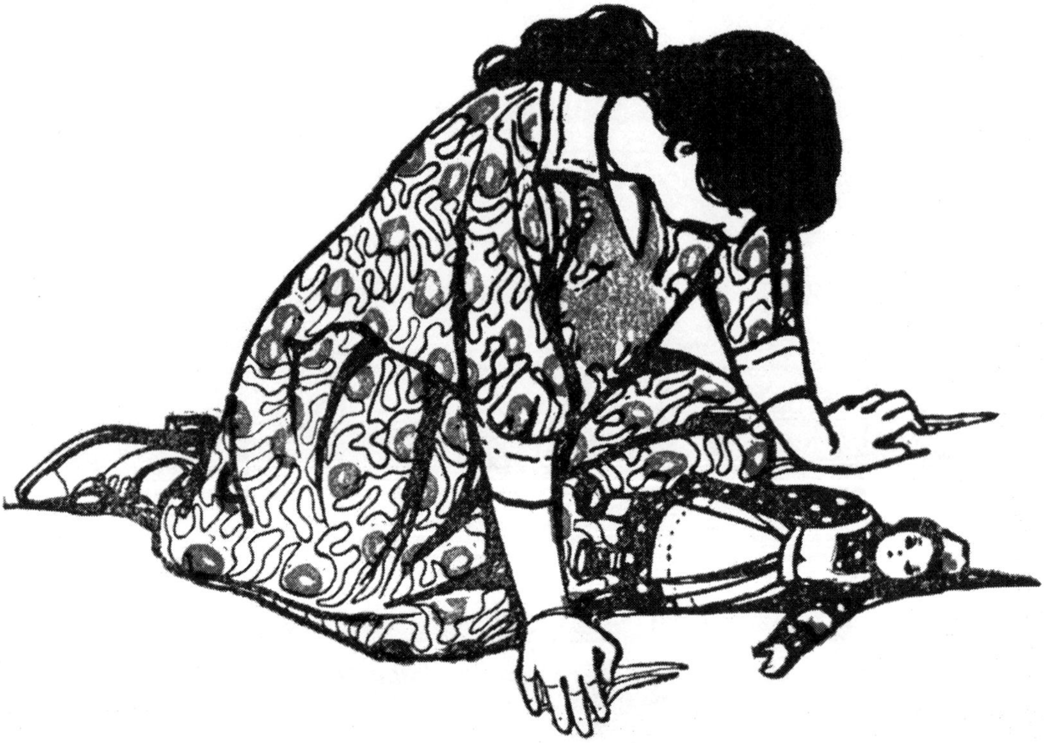

THERE THEY WERE!

"Don't know what you're talking about," pretended Billy.

"Why, Billy!" Mary Frances laughed. "If you will just put a triangular bandage on my hand with your handkerchief, you'll remember."

Billy put it on beautifully, just as you saw it shown on Mary Frances' doll in the picture.

"Now, you remember, Mr. Ambulance Driver!" cried Mary Frances, shaking her finger.

"I don't seem to remember a thing about how I learned," solemnly declared Billy.

"Why, certainly you do. You learned in the Dolls' Hospital," cried Mary Frances.

"Oh, maybe—but don't tell anybody about it, though I must say that a knowledge of bandaging will be most useful when the boy scouts commence their class in advanced first-aid work."

"Will Miss Bossem be their teacher?" teased Mary Frances.

"Aw! Stop talking about that doll of yours dressed up as a nurse, Mary Frances! We boys are beyond the doll-baby age!" Billy walked away in pretended disgust.

"Well," said Mary Frances to herself, "if Billy hadn't known how to put on that bandage I would think I had been dreaming. I know what I'll do! I'll go see if there are any nurses' uniforms in the playroom."

There they were! Each girl doll had one on, just as she wore it at the Fourth of July celebration.

"It must have been real!" concluded Mary Frances. "It must have been! That proves it! Besides, here is Private Brave, and in his wooden hand he is holding the—

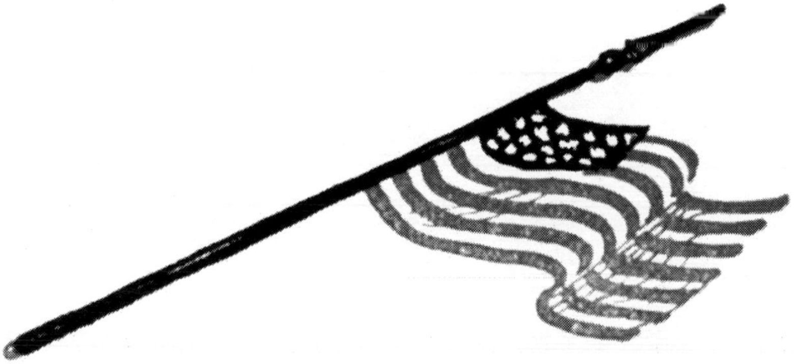

A READY REFERENCE LIST

OF

ORDINARY ACCIDENTS AND ILLNESSES

ALPHABETICALLY ARRANGED

WITH

APPROVED HOME REMEDIES

A FEW GENERAL REMARKS

In the story part of this little book, the author has endeavored to show that success in first-aid treatment of any open wound lies in protecting the wound from infection.

From long years of experience, physicians have found that:

1. Every open wound should be touched with an antiseptic to kill germs which may have entered; and that the best general antiseptic known is iodine.

2. No wound should be closed entirely from the air; therefore, do not use adhesive plaster or collodion to cover a cut or wound, but cover it with sterile gauze after using iodine. The gauze may be held in place at each side by adhesive plaster or by a bandage.

When sending for the doctor, be sure to let him know what is the matter: for instance, poison case, or drowning, or choking—so that he may bring the articles necessary to treat the case.

N. B.—In case of wounds from powder, or punctured wounds, as from rusty nail, see a doctor who will treat patient with anti-tetanic serum.

Read the chapters concerning bandages: Chapters XIII and XVI.

Bandages are used: 1. To hold dressings in place. 2. To support the parts. 3. To hold splints in place.

Never use wet bandages—they shrink in drying.

Never put a tight bandage over a wet compress; use a loose triangular bandage. The exclusion of air might also cause blisters.

An emetic is a medicine which causes vomiting.

To sterilize a needle or knife blade, dip into alcohol or pass through an alcohol or gas flame; or hold in boiling waiter several minutes.

To make a saturated solution dissolve in water as much of the powder mentioned as possible.

NOTE.—Remember that heat in the form of hot drinks and hot applications is the best kind of stimulant.

A READY REFERENCE LIST

Reference to poisonous remedies has been carefully avoided as much as possible.

Where dosage is not mentioned in the following, refer to List of Remedies for the Home Medicine Closet, page 136.

Biliousness.

Give citrate of magnesia, or Epsom or Rochelle salt, or *castor oil. Cracked ice slowly melted in the mouth generally relieves sick stomach.

Hot, clear coffee given after any of the above medicines counteracts greatly the nauseating effect.

Bites of Dogs, Cats, Snakes.

If on a limb, tie a cloth tightly around limb, between wound and body. Loosen slightly in an hour. Encourage bleeding by squeezing, to get poison out, or suck and spit out blood from the wound, being careful to see there are no cuts or wounds in the mouth or lips, through which the poison may enter. *Apply iodine.*

If *hydrophobia* (rabies) is suspected, *send for doctor at once*, who will see that correct treatment is given. This treatment is concerned with the injection of a serum into the blood. See Chapter XVII.

Bites of Insects, Spiders, etc.

Treat as for *stings.*

These are seldom dangerous to life.

"Black Eye."

For "black eye," use either cold or hot water compresses immediately. Massage gently for discoloration.

Bleeding of Gums.

Rinse mouth with alum water—1 teaspoon powdered alum in a glass of ice water; or 1 tsp. tincture of myrrh in 1 tbsp. water.

Blood Blisters.

Do not open. Apply hot water.

*Use one of the proprietary (patent) preparations of castor oil, pleasant to taste.

Broken Bones or Fractures.

There are two kinds of fractures:

1. Simple, where the bone only is broken.
2. Compound, where the skin is broken through at point of fracture.

Treatment:

Send for doctor at once. Much harm is done by unskilled handling. Do not move patient unless absolutely necessary.

If a compound fracture, apply iodine. Bandage a sterile gauze compress loosely over wound, tie a cloth tightly around limb, between wound and body. See "Hemorrhage" in this list.

Using *extreme gentleness*, place limb in comfortable position on a pillow or pad, and tie fast with strips of muslin or bandages.

If impossible to get doctor for a long time, and patient must be moved, use extreme carefulness, and tie limb to padded splints with bandages.

Rulers, umbrellas, sticks, rolled newspapers, may be used for splints. If an arm, after applying splints, place in sling made with triangular bandage, or pin coat sleeve to front of shirt.

Treat for "Shock."

Bruises or Contusions.

"Black and blue" spots from blow or fall or pinching, causing blood vessels to rupture under skin.

Apply at first:

Ice, or ice water; or
Alcohol and water, half and half; or
Witch hazel, or arnica; or
Vinegar diluted with water.

Afterward use hot applications. Gentle rubbing or massaging helps dispel the discoloration. If surface is scraped, as from fall in sand, see "Wounds."

Burns and Scalds.

There are three different degrees of burns:

1. Mere reddening of the skin (slight burns).
2. Formation of blisters (deeper burns).
3. Charring and destruction of the skin and tissues.

1. For slight burns (first degree), apply any of the following:

Bicarbonate of soda (baking soda) mixed in water to the thickness of milk, olive oil, cream, vaseline, lard, butter, white of egg, or flour and water paste, or starch and water.

Spread gauze compress* with the material used, and bandage loosely in place.

2. In deeper burns (second degree), be careful in removing clothing—cut it off, if necessary, to prevent tearing the skin.

Bandage on loosely compresses wet in one of the following:

(*a*) Normal Salt Solution (1 level tsp. salt in 1 pint boiled water);

or

(*b*) Carron Oil (½ lime water, ½ linseed oil);

or

(*c*) Saturated Solution Bicarbonate of Soda. (Dissolve as much baking soda as possible in a cup of boiled water;)

or

(*d*) Picric Acid Gauze Compress.

Follow any of these treatments with Boric Acid Ointment. (See List of Medicines, No. 22).

Blisters. Later, puncture blisters near base with a sharp instrument which has been sterilized by dipping in alcohol. Mop up the watery discharge with a little aseptic absorbent cotton, throwing it away. Never open blisters far enough to loosen skin. Dress with gauze compresses, dusted with boric acid. Use several small compresses if burned surface is large.

3. In very severe burns (third degree) little can be done. *Send for the doctor.* Do not remove clothing. Make patient as comfortable as possible.

For burns about the eye, anoint with olive oil and wash out with boric acid solution in eye dropper or eye cup. (See List of Medicines, No. 3.) Use compresses wrung out of ice water. See doctor.

Car Sickness.

Fresh air. Lying-down position.

Do not look out of window at moving objects. Keep eyes closed.

Chilblains.

Chilblains are the result of too rapid warming of cold parts, generally feet or fingers. Sometimes for years after being frost-bitten, exposure to severe cold will produce itching and burning, and perhaps swelling and ulcers.

Treatment:

Rub with turpentine or alcohol. The rubbing in itself is excellent. See doctor.

*A compress is several thicknesses of gauze or other clean material

Chills.

Use heat. Apply hot-water bags under arms, on thighs and at feet. Give hot foot bath, in which is 1 tbsp. mustard. Rub limbs toward body, to restore circulation. Give hot coffee or tea, or hot lemonade. Wrap in blankets and put to bed. Chills indicate oncoming illness—see doctor! See Chapter XI.

Choking.

Slap on back. Pass finger down throat. This usually causes vomiting. If a child, hold him up by the feet, head downward, and slap on the back. Send for doctor, if severe.

Coal Gas, Suffocation from.

Send for doctor.

Get patient into fresh air—loosen clothing. Keep patient warm with hot-water bags. Rub limbs toward body. Dash cold water in face. Doctor will probably use artificial respiration.

Colds.

At the *first sign* of "taking a cold"—use some simple remedy, such as inhaling camphor from time to time for several hours. Dampen the center of a handkerchief in water, and drop on it some spirit of camphor. *Eat a sliced onion.**

Take two drops of spirit of camphor on a tsp. sugar.

Or, drop five drops camphor in ½ tumbler of water. Take a tsp. every half hour.

Ginger tea is a much valued old-fashioned remedy. Pour boiling water over a tbsp. bruised ginger root. Let stand two hours. The dose is 1 tbsp. every hour or two.

If the "cold" continues, take a laxative, such as castor oil or rhubarb, and follow the dose with a hot foot bath at night and hot lemonade after getting into bed, to induce perspiration. Keep well covered.

If a cough comes with the cold, lemon juice and sugar syrup make a pleasant cough remedy; or molasses-and-vinegar syrup is liked by children. Mix in the proportion of 1 tbsp. vinegar to 2 tbsp. molasses.

Flaxseed tea will sometimes relieve a "tickling" cough. Pour 2 cups of boiling water over 1 tbsp. whole flaxseeds. Stir; let simmer gently one-half hour. Add juice of half a lemon, and sugar if desired. Take a tbsp. as often as wished.

If the chest is sore, rub it with camphorated oil, or ammonia liniment, which is made by shaking together in a bottle 4 tbsp. olive (sweet) oil and 1 tbsp. household ammonia. This hardens upon standing a few days—so it is best made as needed.

*If to the onion is added a tbsp. or two of water, a tbsp. vinegar (and olive oil, if desired), pepper and salt, it will be found a palatable salad with bread and butter, and will be liked by most children.

All these are simple home remedies, but if a cold is severe, see a doctor. A neglected cold is dangerous.

Colic.

Colic pains in abdomen are generally caused by indigestible food, overeating, constipation, etc.

Treatment:

Give peppermint in hot water; hot-water enema. Keep abdomen warmly wrapped in flannel; use hot-water bottles, or turpentine stupe.

If a child—massage abdomen with warm olive oil.

Convulsions of Children.

Caused by indigestion, constipation or oncoming illness. Child becomes stiff, pulse is weak and rapid. Breathing is feeble, face is pale at first, afterward livid.

Treatment:

Send for doctor. Place child in warm bath, with ice bag (or ice-water cloths) on head.

Corns.

For soft corn, apply vaseline.

For hard corn, apply iodine and remove pressure by using corn plaster.

For a very sore corn, use a bread poultice at night.

Croup.

Croup is generally more alarming than dangerous.

Give 1 teaspoon syrup of ipecac to make child vomit.

Apply cloths wrung out of hot water on neck and chest.

A boiling tea kettle, in which there are 2 tbsp. compound tincture of benzoin, will afford relief. Direct the steam toward the child so that some of it may be inhaled.

Keep the child in the same warm room forty-eight hours, maintaining the atmosphere at an even temperature.

The day after the attack, give the child castor oil or simple syrup of rhubarb.

If croup does not clear up in twenty-four hours, see the doctor for membranous croup or diphtheria.

Cuts (Slight).

Touch with—

Tincture of iodine, or if iodine is not at hand,

Alcohol, or

Vinegar and water—equal parts.

If edges are spread far apart, strap together with narrow strips of adhesive plaster across wound. Wrap with sterile gauze.

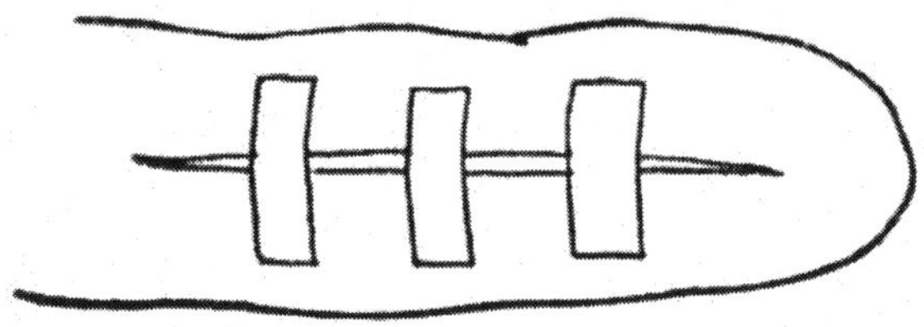

HOW TO STRAP A CUT FINGER

If cut is larger, after applying iodine, fasten on a gauze compress—cut ½ inch larger than wound—with a bandage, or with strips of adhesive plaster.

Caution.—Never cover a wound or cut airtight. (See also Chapter VII.)

Diarrhea.

Usually caused by indigestion, impure water, etc. Home remedies are raw flour and water paste; a raw egg in a cup of hot tea; spiced syrup of rhubarb.

Give a dose of castor oil to clear the digestive tract of the irritating material. If there is much pain, keep abdomen warm with flannel and hot-water bag. If a small child, restrict diet to barley water and white of egg in water.

Give adults milk and other liquid foods. If persistent, see doctor.

Earache.

Caused sometimes by bad teeth, but generally by cold or hardened ear wax.

Hold ear over cloth wrung out of hot water, on which are several drops of alcohol. Syringe ear with warm bicarbonate of soda water—1 tsp. to a cup; or peroxide of hydrogen water—1 tbsp. to a cup of water.

One drop laudanum, or one drop arnica to three drops very warm olive oil, dropped into ear with a medicine dropper, often relieves pain; or cotton may be saturated with the warm olive oil and placed in the ear and covered with dry cotton. To prevent hardening of wax: keep ear anointed with ordinary red vaseline (unbleached vaseline). For watery discharge of ear, dust with dry boric acid.

Fainting.

Caused by too small a quantity of blood to the brain.

To prevent: Fresh air; drink of cold water; ½ tsp. aromatic spirit of ammonia in water; bending head over between knees.

If the person has fainted:

Keep crowd back; place in lying-down position.

Dash face with cold water.

Let patient inhale smelling salts or household ammonia.

Rub limbs toward body.

Remember: An unconscious person cannot swallow. Medicine may enter windpipe and cause strangulation. After patient becomes conscious, give stimulants; such as aromatic spirit of ammonia or hot coffee.

Fever Blisters (Cold Sores).

Apply boric acid ointment,* or touch frequently with spirit of nitre or spirit of camphor.

Fits.

There are two kinds:

1. *Hysterical*—sobbing, crying and laughing without cause, jerky movement of the limbs.

Treatment:

Let patient quietly alone.

2. *Epileptic*—convulsive movements and unconsciousness.

Treatment:

Keep patient from biting tongue by putting a piece of wood or folded cloth between teeth. Lay on side; loosen clothing; turn face to side so that secretions may not strangle.

After the fit, let patient sleep.

Do *not* give stimulants.

Foreign Body in Ear.

If an insect, drown out with warm olive oil, or pour a little pure alcohol into ear.

Do not probe ear.

Foreign Body in Eye.

Wink. Do not rub.

Lift upper lid down over lower, blowing opposite nostril.

If these means fail, turn lid back over a toothpick, removing foreign body gently with the pointed corner of a handkerchief. For bits of plaster, use dilute vinegar in eye cup. For acids, use very dilute bicarbonate of soda solution. (See Chapter XI.)

Frost Bites.

Parts frozen turn whitish or waxy looking.

Do not bring patient into a warm room.

Use cold applications. Keep in cold room. (See Chapter VII.)

Rub with snow or ice-water cloths, *very gradually* applying heat.

"Gum Boils" or "Canker Sores."

*See list of Medicines No. 22.

So-called "gum boils" or "canker sores" are little ulcer-like sores which at times appear in children's mouths, caused by disarrangement of the stomach. Local applications, such as borax or powdered alum, shrink the sores and give a little relief; but the child should be given a dose of calcined magnesia at night or citrate of magnesia in the morning. (Never give a small dose of citrate of magnesia; a child of twelve years should take a tumblerful.)

Heat Exhaustion. (Collapse Due to Excessive Heat.) Dangerous!

In heat exhaustion, the symptoms and treatment are similar to *shock*: pale face; weak, feeble heart beats; great weakness, but not unconsciousness; shallow breathing; cold, clammy perspiration on face.

Treatment: Send for doctor. Remove to cool place.

Do *not* use cold applications. Give stimulants—hot coffee, tea, aromatic spirit of ammonia, etc. Cover with blankets and use hot-water bottles.

Hemorrhage (Severe Bleeding).

Send for doctor. While waiting, try to staunch flow of blood.

If wound is in a limb:

If blood is *red*, and comes in *spurts* (*arterial*)—

Elevate wounded part, tie cloth tightly around limb between wound and body, or use a tourniquet,* loosening it in one hour. If not loosened, there is danger of gangrene.

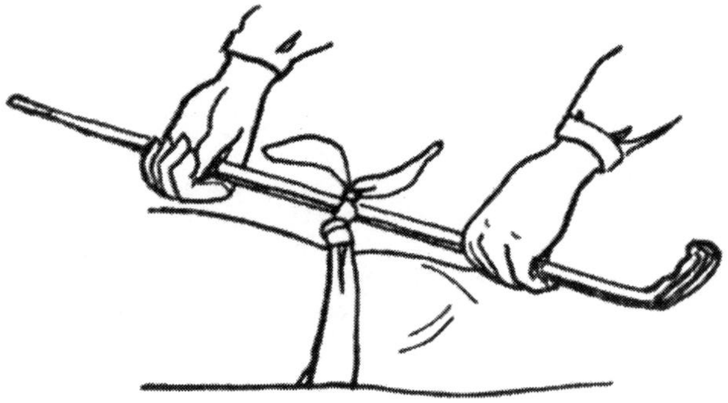

USING A TOURNIQUET

If blood is *dark*, and comes in slow flow (venous)—

Tie a cloth around between *end* of limb and wound. Or use a tourniquet, loosening it in one hour.

In either case, bandage a clean gauze compress against wound. If unable to use these methods because of too rapid bleeding, press fingers into wound, but have another person tie as described. Do not use finger pressure if possible to avoid, for the wound should be kept clean.

Any of the following tend to stop bleeding:

Ice or ice water.

*A tourniquet (pronounced turn-e-ket) is a constricting band used to stop bleeding. Usually a triangular bandage is folded into cravat form and tied loosely about the limb; then twisted as shown in this picture. A rubber band, necktie, garter or a piece of rope may be used in emergency.

Very hot water.

Vinegar, 1 tbsp. to 4 tbsp. water.

Salt, 1 tsp. to 4 tbsp. water.

Wet a compress (several thicknesses of gauze) in any of these and bandage on wound.

For hemorrhage of lungs, place ice-bag on chest.

DO NOT GIVE WHISKEY OR BRANDY!

For slight wounds, see "*Cuts*."

Hiccough.

Generally caused by indigestion.

Nine to fifteen swallows of water without taking a breath, or one or two soda-mint tablets, will generally give relief. If persistent, cause vomiting by tickling throat with fingers, or by swallowing a cup of warm water in which ½ tsp. mustard is dissolved. (See Chapter XI.)

Hives (Nettle Rash).

For itching, rub into them common table salt, or bathe with equal parts vinegar and water.

Hives indicate stomach trouble. Give citrate of magnesia.

If hives persist, give ½ tsp. table salt in water or ¼ tsp. cream of tartar in ¼ glass of water three times a day for three days.

If hives still persist, consult doctor. (See Chapter X.)

Indigestion.

Hot water. Soda mints. Aromatic spirit of ammonia. Bicarbonate of soda (baking soda). Hot applications to the stomach.

Itching.

For itching which affects the whole body, give a bath; apply sulphur ointment.

Sulphur ointment is made by rubbing 2 tbsp. flowers of sulphur into a dessert-spoonful of lard.

Lice in Hair (Pediculosis).

Wash hair with kerosene, leaving it on over night; or use tincture of *larkspur** in the same way.

Perhaps the best remedy is *fishberries*.*

Five cents worth of the berries may be boiled in 1 pint water for ten minutes.

Wash hair next day after using any of these remedies.

*Poison.

Nails (Ingrowing).

Scrape surface—a piece of glass is good for this purpose. Cut in V-shape. Pack absorbent cotton under affected side. Paint with iodine.

Nausea (Sick Stomach).

Give small bits of cracked ice. Soda mint. Lime water.

To crack ice: wrap a piece in a cloth, and hammer.

Nosebleed.

Head in upright position. Raise arm on bleeding side. Loosen collar. Apply ice in a cloth to bridge of nose and back of neck. A roll of paper under upper lip. Snuff cold tea up nose, or salt water, 1 tsp. to cup water, or the same of powdered alum.

If bleeding continues, tie a small wad of cotton with thread; dip it into peroxide of hydrogen, and plug nostril by pushing the cotton gently with a pencil. The thread is used to withdraw cotton.

If these means fail, send for doctor.

Perspiration.

For deodorizing—use a paste of borax and water.

Poison Ivy Rash.

The poison ivy plant has three leaves in clusters.

Do not scratch.* Mop on rash a saturated solution of Epsom salt (as much as can be dissolved in a cup of water); or, wash with saturated solution boric acid. Allow it to dry in the air.

Lime water may be used in place of boric acid.

Wash the affected surface every day, dry and repeat treatment.

Sweet fern tea is very good. Steep the sweet fern in boiling water an hour, and apply to rash.

Poisoning—Treatment and Antidotes.

Send for doctor, but work immediately.

If you do not know what caused the poisoning, make patient vomit as soon as possible by giving 1 tsp. mustard in a cup of warm water, or 1 tsp. salt in a cup of warm water, or 2 tsp. ipecac. Repeat if necessary.

After vomiting, give white of egg stirred in water; milk; or boiled starch. Give hot coffee as stimulant.

*Mothers who find it difficult to keep children from scratching this rash at night may cover hands with small triangular bandages.

There are three divisions of poisons:

(a) Those that affect the nervous system; as opium, aconite, alcohol.

(b) Those that irritate; as arsenic, tainted food.

(c) Those that corrode (burn); as carbolic acid, oxalic acid, bichloride of mercury (which is corrosive sublimate), lye, caustic alkalies.

In any case of poisoning, remember that the first-aid treatment is to—

1. Remove the poisonous material, or
2. Neutralize its further action.
3. Remedy the ill effects already produced.

1. To remove the poison, give emetic (to produce vomiting); as mustard and water or ipecac or salt and water.

An emetic is *not usually used, however, in corrosive poisoning* (see (c) above) except in the case of bichloride of mercury, for which see special direction below.

2. To neutralize the further effect of poison, give something to destroy its action; for instance, if lye is swallowed, give dilute acid, as vinegar and water.

3. To remedy the ill effects, give stimulants; as strong coffee.

Some Antidotes

For Carbolic Acid.—In case of poisoning from carbolic acid, give alcohol and water; or, if alcohol is not at hand, 1 tbsp. Epsom salt in a glass of water, or beaten whites of eggs in milk. Use hot-water bottle.

Treatment of Poisoning from Any Other Acids than Carbolic (Corrosives).—Give alkalies—baking soda, 1 tsp. in a cup water. Lime water, magnesia, whitewash diluted with water; even a tbsp. of strong soapsuds. Follow with beaten white of egg and milk, olive oil, coffee.

Treatment of Poisoning from Alkalies (Lye, Household Ammonia, etc.). (*Corrosives.*) Do not cause vomiting. 1 tbsp. vinegar in a cup of water; lemon juice and water, half and half; orange juice; follow with whites of egg in milk, olive oil; flour and water; hot coffee.

For Bichloride of Mercury (Corrosive Sublimate).—Give beaten whites of eggs in water; emetic—warm mustard water (1 tsp. to cup); hot coffee. Keep patient warm.

For Iodine.—Give boiled starch, or starch and water, or flour and water. Give hot coffee. Keep patient warm.

For Arsenic (*Irritant. See (b).*).—Give an emetic; tincture of iron, white of eggs, coffee.

For Laudanum (*Affects Nerves. See (a).*).—Keep patient awake by walking. Give strong black coffee.

Powder Wounds.

Dangerous because powder carries germs of "lockjaw."

Wash the skin. Paint with iodine.

Apply vaseline. This loosens any bits of powder, which may be washed off the next day.

Absolutely every wound of this character must be treated by a doctor, who will inject anti-tetanic serum.(See Chapter XII.)

Prickly Heat.

Rash, especially on young children, caused by heat. Wash with warm water and soap. Apply alcohol (one part to three of water). Dust with talcum powder. (See Chapter X.)

Ptomaine Poisoning.

Symptoms: Severe nausea, purging diarrhea. See doctor.

Treatment: Vomiting is necessary. Give cup warm water in which 1 tsp. mustard is dissolved, or give 2 tsp. ipecac. Give castor oil.

Apply external heat—hot-water bags.

Give 1 tsp. paregoric, if you have it.

Sea-Sickness.

Cracked ice. The best preventive is to see the doctor a week before going on ocean trip.

Shock.

The word "shock" refers to the condition of nervous depression which follows any accident, or sometimes the sight of one's own wound. The breathing is feeble; the face pale. Send for doctor. Place patient in lying-down position. Use hot-water bottles. Give hot coffee; aromatic spirit of ammonia. Gently massage or rub limbs toward body.

Keep body covered and warm. (Sec Chapter III.)

Sore Throat.

At night wrap a cloth wet in alcohol around outside of throat. Gargle with salt and water (1 tsp. to a glass), or borax and water in same proportion, or hot tea, or with the following—

Gargle:

2 tbsp. vinegar,

1 tbsp. salt,

Water to fill a tumbler.

If persistent, see doctor.

Splinters.

Open wound with sterile needle. Pull splinter out from the direction it entered. Apply iodine or turpentine.

If under nail, cut nail in V-shape at point where splinter entered, before extracting splinter. Use tweezers. Paint the place with iodine.

A pair of extracting tweezers cost little, and should be in every household.

To make needle or tweezers sterile, dip in alcohol or pass through a flame.

Sprain.

If at all severe, send for doctor.

Elevate limb. Apply cloth wrung from ice water, or an ice bag, for several hours, then apply heat. Bandage to keep limb at rest.

Stiff Neck.

Rub with sassafras oil or with capsicum vaseline.

Stings.

Extract sting if it remains imbedded in flesh. Apply household ammonia, diluted with a little water, or solution of bicarbonate of soda (1 tsp. soda to 1 cup water).

Mud, wet salt, slice of onion, arnica, witch hazel, camphor are soothing. If there is much swelling, apply cracked ice. Apply spirit of camphor or alcohol to mosquito bites.

Strain of Muscles.

Apply ice-water cloths or an ice bag. If the cold fails to give relief in an hour, apply heat. Bathe with arnica, alcohol and water, and rest the parts.

Sunburn.

To prevent: Anoint exposed parts with cold cream, vaseline, or use toilet powder before going out.

Treatment: Never wash sunburn. Never open blisters.

Apply—

1 part lime water, 3 parts olive oil, shaken together in a bottle.

Sunstroke (Collapse Due to Exposure to Rays of Sun).

Distinguish between sunstroke and heat exhaustion.

In sunstroke the symptoms are: red face; rapid heart beats; headache; vomiting; fever; noisy breathing and sighing; stupor; no perspiration; unconsciousness.

Treatment: Send for doctor. Remove to cool place. Loosen clothing. Apply ice in a cloth, or cloths wrung out of ice water to entire body.

Give NO STIMULANTS—NO WHISKEY OR BRANDY.

Toothache.

See dentist.

Hot applications. Iodine painted on gums. Oil of cloves on cotton in tooth. (Be careful in using this.) (See Chapter XI.)

Warts.

Apply a "corn cure" containing "cannabis indica." Nitric acid may be applied, but it is so dangerous a poison that it is unsafe for children to handle.

Wounds.

See "*Hemorrhage*" for deep, bleeding wounds.

If surface is scraped, as from a fall in sand, wash wound with hot water (which has been boiled) and pure soap, such as Castile, and paint with iodine. Fasten a sterile gauze compress in place over scraped surface with a bandage or adhesive plaster.

See also "Cuts," "Powder Wounds."

PLASTERS, POULTICES AND STUPES

Moist heat, in the form of plasters, poultices, and stupes, is more penetrating than dry heat, and is often employed in cases of severe inflammation.

Mustard plasters are in such common use that it seems unnecessary to mention their value as counter-irritants.

To Make a Mustard Plaster.—For an adult, mix together in the proportion of 1 tbsp. mustard and 3 or 4 tbsp. flour, and rub into a smooth paste with *warm* water—not *hot* or *cold* water.

For a child, use from 4 to 6 tbsp. flour to ½ tbsp. mustard.

Spread the paste on muslin, turning each edge over about an inch. Cover with gauze or a piece of thin muslin.

To prevent blistering, it is well to add beaten white of egg in making the plaster, and to anoint the skin with vaseline or olive oil before applying the plaster.

After removing plaster (in about fifteen minutes), cover skin with thin muslin.

If much inflamed, apply olive oil or vaseline.

Flaxseed is the favorite material for making a poultice, because the oil in the seed retains heat longer than most other materials.

To Make a Flaxseed Poultice.—Into a cup of boiling water, stir as much ground flaxseed as it will "take up." Spread on muslin; fold edges over one inch or more, and cover with one layer of gauze. Poultice is applied as hot as possible to the surface. Replace in one hour.

A bread poultice is made by laying a slice of bread in a sieve, and pouring hot water over it. It is placed on muslin and applied direct.

Poultices are not used as much as they were a number of years ago, but stupes give such relief to pain in the abdomen that mention should be made of the

Turpentine Stupe.—To 1 pint boiling water, add 2 tsp. oil of turpentine. Dip a large piece of flannel into this. Wring out by twisting in a towel—lay wet flannel in center of towel, fold edges of towel over the flannel and twist ends of towel until the flannel is quite dry. Apply hot! Cover with a large dry towel. Watch that it does not blister. Anoint with vaseline or olive oil before applying stupe if skin is very sensitive.

An easier method is to mix together equal parts oil of turpentine and olive oil. Heat by setting the cup containing the mixture in very hot water. Apply by rubbing. Cover with woolen cloth wrung out of hot water, as described above.

LIST OF REMEDIES FOR THE HOME MEDICINE CLOSET

In every home there should be a certain closet or shelf high above *little* children's reach, where the medicines and articles needed in emergencies are kept. Among these should be found, plainly labeled, the following:

1. Tincture of Iodine.
2. Aromatic Spirit of Ammonia.
3. Boric Acid Powder.
4. Stearate of Zinc.
5. Pure Alcohol.
6. Lime Water.
7. Carron Oil.T
8. Epsom Salt.
9. Soda-Mint-and-Pepsin Tablets.
10. Baking Soda.
11. Household Ammonia.
12. Adhesive (Zinc Oxide) Plaster.
13. Tube Vaseline.
14. Capsicum Vaseline.
15. Peroxide of Hydrogen.
16. Castor Oil.
17. Witch Hazel.
18. Essence of Ginger.
19. Syrup of Ipecac.
20. Spirit of Camphor.
21. Sweet Spirit of Nitre.
22. Boric Acid Ointment.
23. Powdered Alum.
24. Borax.
25. Spiced Syrup of Rhubarb.
26. Picric Acid Gauze.
27. Aromatic Smelling Salts.
28. Oil of Cloves.
29. Normal Salt Solution.
30. Powdered Mustard.
31. Essence of Peppermint.
32. Tincture of Arnica.
33. Oil of Turpentine.
34. Aseptic Absorbent Cotton.
35. Sterile Gauze.
36. Triangular Bandages.
37. Roller Bandages.
38. Rubber Ear Syringe.
39. Fountain Syringe.
40. Measuring Glass.
41. Eye Dropper.
42. Hot-Water Bottle.

For description of the above remedies and dosage, see the following pages.

Important Note.—All bottles containing medicines which are poisonous when swallowed, such as iodine, should be labeled with red ink and should be tied with a rag about the neck, in order that even in the dark, no mistake may be made.

Read labels three times before giving or taking medicine:

Before taking from closet;

Before measuring dose;

Before giving to patient.

Have amount given for a dose written on each label.

MEASURES.

30 drops	½ tsp. (teaspoon)
60 drops	1 tsp., or 1 dram.
2 tsp.	1 dessertspoon.
4 tsp.	1 tbsp. (tablespoon)
1 tbsp.	½ ounce.
2 tbsp.	1 ounce.

1. Tincture of Iodine.

(One ounce in a large-mouthed glass-stoppered bottle.)

This should be in every household and every member above ten years of age should know where it is kept. Any open wound or cut should be immediately touched with this antiseptic.

Iodine is a *poison* if swallowed, but is the best household remedy in cases of cuts or wounds. It should be applied to such injuries immediately, for it destroys germs. Iodine may be applied direct by pouring on wound; or with a small wad of absorbent cotton fastened to a toothpick.

If iodine is swallowed by accident, give cornstarch and water, or boiled starch, or bread softened in water.

To take iodine stains out of materials, use strong household ammonia.

2. Aromatic Spirit of Ammonia.

(One ounce in glass-stoppered bottle.)

Dose:

Children, 10 drops in ¼ glass of water.

Grown people, ½ tsp. in ¼ glass of water.

Dose may be safely repeated every hour for several hours.

This is used for nervousness, headaches, indigestion, fainting, etc.

(Remember that an unconscious person cannot swallow, so do not give an unconscious person medicine, for it may cause choking.)

3. Boric Acid Powder.

(One-half pound.)

Boric acid is not an acid, but a simple harmless alkali.

Useful in solution as a mouth wash; also for stings and for sore eyes. Dissolve as much as possible in a cup of freshly boiled water. For sore eyes, use in an eye-dropper or an eye-cup. It is both harmless and safe. Sometimes the dry powder is dusted on the blistered surface of a burn to dry blisters. Talcum powders contain a great deal of boric acid, which is cooling and healing.

4. Compound Stearate of Zinc.

(One ounce.)

A simple, excellent dusting powder for skin irritations.

5. Pure Alcohol.

(One pint in glass-stoppered bottle. The glass stopper prevents evaporation.)

Useful for bathing in case of fever—to reduce temperature. Dip needle into alcohol before taking a splinter out—to "sterilize" or remove germs from needle. If iodine becomes too strong because of evaporation, add a little pure alcohol.

NOTE.—"Wood" alcohol is a poison, sometimes causing blindness; even used for bathing, it injures the eyes.

"Denatured" alcohol is a poison.

6. Lime Water.

(Five cents' worth.)

Dose: 1 to 2 tbsp. or more in water or milk.

Used for acid indigestion, for poisoning from acids, and in making carron oil.

7. Carron Oil.

(One-half pint.)

Carron oil is excellent for burns. It may be purchased at the drug store, or made by shaking together in a bottle equal parts of linseed oil and lime water; for instance: one-quarter cup linseed oil, one quarter cup lime water.

8. Epsom Salt.

(One-half pound.)

Useful as a laxative.

Dose: 1 tsp. to 1 tbsp. in a glass of water.

To relieve the skin in ivy poisoning, dissolve as much Epsom salt as possible in a quarter cup boiled water. When cool, bathe skin and allow to dry in the air.

9. Soda-Mint-and-Pepsin Tablets.

A simple remedy for indigestion.

10. Baking Soda (Bicarbonate of Soda).

(Two ounces in a box or glass.)

Useful in solution in case of scalds or burns, and stings of insects.

For indigestion: dose ½ tsp. in ½ glass hot water.

11. Household Ammonia.

(Label, "POISON.")

In case of fainting, hold a little distance from patient's nose. Useful for stings of insects.

12. Adhesive (Zinc Oxide) Plaster.

(One yard, one-half inch wide.)

Useful for holding dressings in place or for fastening end of bandages, etc.; for support in sprains in place of bandages; for strapping a cut, but should *not* be used to *cover* a cut or wound.

13. Tube Vaseline.

Useful for burns, chapped hands, granulated eyelids. Do *not* put vaseline on *fresh* cuts or wounds.

If a glass stopper is oiled with vaseline, it will not "stick" fast.

14. Tube Capsicum Vaseline.

Used for stiff neck, and in place of mustard plaster when only a mild irritant is needed.

15. Peroxide of Hydrogen.

(Four ounces.)

Do not use on cuts! Cotton saturated with peroxide of hydrogen will generally stop severe nosebleed. Used sometimes for burns. Keep bottle in a *dark* closet; it deteriorates in the light.

Note.—Peroxide of hydrogen is recommended by State Boards of Health as a protection against Infantile Paralysis. Use as a spray for nose and throat, or as a gargle, in the proportion of one part peroxide to three parts water.

16. Castor Oil.

(Two ounces.)

Dose: Children, 1 to 2 tsp.; adults, 1 to 2 tbsp.

A mild purgative, clearing the intestines of undigested food in case of acute indigestion.

It may be given in capsules; or one of the patent ("proprietary") preparations may be given. There are one or two of these which are not at all unpleasant to take. An easy method of taking castor oil: hold a piece of ice in the mouth before taking; and after, rinse the mouth with ice water.

17. Witch Hazel.

(Ten cents' worth.)

For sprains, stings, bites of insects.

Best applied in wet compress.

18. Essence, or Tincture, or Spirit of (Jamaica) Ginger.

(One ounce.)

Dose: ½ tsp. in a tbsp. hot water. Less for children.

For colic and indigestion.

19. Syrup of Ipecac.

(Two ounces.)

Dose: As expectorant, 5 to 10 drops; as emetic, 1 tsp. to 1 tbsp., according to age.

Used as an emetic—to produce vomiting—in croup, in cases of poisoning, etc.

Useful in small doses in bronchitis and asthma.

20. Spirit of Camphor.

(Two ounces.)

This may be made by pouring pure alcohol on pure gum camphor.

It is useful for colds when they first appear. Dose: 2 drops on a tsp. sugar.

Excellent for mosquito bites.

21. Sweet Spirit of Nitre.

(Two ounces.)

Dose:

Children, 3 to 10 drops in ¼ glass of water.

Adults, 20 drops to 1 tsp. in ¼ glass of water.

For fever and colds. Apply to fever blisters (cold sores) to allay inflammation.

22. Boric Acid Ointment.

Excellent for fever blisters (cold sores). Made by rubbing 1 tbsp. boric acid powder into 1 tsp. vaseline.

23. Powdered Alum.

(One ounce.)

Useful for bleeding gums, canker spots, as a gargle in sore throat, etc.

Dissolve a tsp. in a glass of water.

24. Borax.

(One pound.)

Useful as a gargle or mouth wash—one tsp. in a glass of water; or as a deodorant of perspiration, and for general cleansing purposes.

25. Spiced Syrup of Rhubarb.

(Two ounces.)

Dose:

Children ½ to 1 tsp.

Adults 2 tsp.

For pain in abdomen, indigestion, diarrhea.

26. Picric Acid Gauze.

(One small package.)

This is excellent as a compress for burns, but it leaves a stain on clothing which cannot be removed.

27. Aromatic Smelling Salts.

Inhaled for faintness, headache, etc.

28. Oil of Cloves.

(One-half ounce.)

For toothache. Saturate a piece of cotton and pack in the tooth after cleaning out the cavity. Cover with dry cotton.

29. Normal Salt Solution.

Excellent for burns.

To make: Add 1 level tsp. table salt to 1 pint water which has boiled 20 minutes. Do not use more salt than directions call for.

30. Mustard (Powdered).

(One-quarter pound.)

One tsp. in a glass of lukewarm water will cause vomiting. Useful as an emetic in cases of poisoning, and in form of mustard plaster.

31. Essence of Peppermint.

(Two ounces.)

Dose:

Children, 3 to 10 drops in ¼ glass of water.

Adults, 10 to 20 drops in ¼ glass of water.

For colic, flatulence (gas), heart-burn.

Sometimes used externally for slight burns.

32. Tincture of Arnica.

(Four ounces.)

Applied externally as a remedy for strains, sprains, and bruises.

33. Oil of Turpentine.

(Two ounces.)

Useful for chilblains, and in "stupes." See Ready Reference List, page 136.

(Buy this at the drug store—it is not the kind used in paint.)

34. Aseptic (Sterile) Absorbent Cotton.

(Small package.)

"Aseptic" means clean, or free from germs. Keep clean in package, opening end only as needed. Throw away all used cotton.

35. Sterile Gauze.

(Buy a one-yard package at the drug store. Keep it wrapped.)

"Sterile" means clean in a medical sense—free from germs. Do not handle. Hands are seldom clean in a medical sense. Never use old rags or pieces of handkerchiefs unless freshly laundered, but if possible use sterile gauze for wrapping cuts or wounds.

36. Triangular Bandages.

The triangular bandage is the bandage used for first-aid emergencies.

The roller bandages are for more permanent use.

It is most convenient to have on hand one of the Red Cross First Aid Outfits, the contents of which are so packed as to keep them free from dust.

The simplest of these outfits contains all material necessary in ordinary household accidents:

A triangular muslin bandage.

A gauze bandage.

Two safety pins.

On the triangular bandage are printed pictures showing the way in which it is used. (See Chapter XIII.)

To a gauze bandage a pad of gauze is sewed. This pad may be tied over a wound without being touched with the hands.

The safety pins are to hold bandages in place, but a stitch is better.

37. Roller Bandages.

In addition to the above, in every medicine closet there should be:

Three gauze roller bandages, 1 inch wide (for bandaging fingers).

Three gauze roller bandages, 2½ inches wide (for bandaging arms, etc.).

It is best to buy roller bandages, wrapped ready for use, at the drug store. Never use a wet bandage, for it shrinks as it dries, and stops free circulation of the blood. (See Chapter XVI.)

38. Rubber Ear Syringe.

39. Fountain Syringe.

40. Graduate Measuring Glass, marked with dosage—teaspoonful, tablcspoonful.

glass with markings on side

41. Eye Dropper, which can be used to drop medicine.

dropper

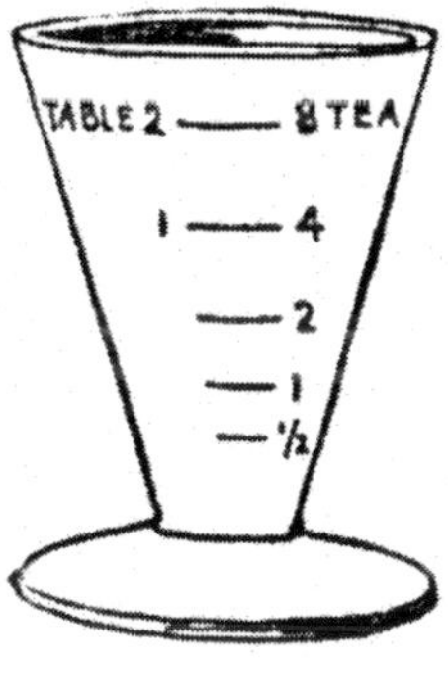

GRADUATE MEASURING GLASS

EYE DROPPER

42. Hot-Water Bottle.

While this list of contents of the Home Medicine Closet may seem long, the cost is but little, and the timely use of some of the remedies may prevent serious illness and save doctors' bills.

Made in the USA
Monee, IL
04 November 2026

67380845R00072